Contents

Note on References

References in the text within square brackets relate to the numbered items in the Select Bibliography, followed, where necessary, by the page number in italics, for example [1:*45*].

Disease, Medicine and Society in England 1550–1860

Prepared for
The Economic History Society by

ROY PORTER

Senior Lecturer in the History of Medicine,
Wellcome Institute for the
History of Medicine,
London

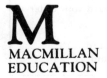

**MACMILLAN
EDUCATION**

First published 1987

Published by
Higher and Further Education Division
MACMILLAN PUBLISHERS LTD
Houndmills, Basingstoke, Hampshire RG21 2XS
and London
Companies and representatives
throughout the world

Printed in Hong Kong

British Library Cataloguing in Publication Data
Porter, Roy, 1946–
Disease, medicine and society in England,
1550–1860.—(Studies in economic and
social history)
1. Social medicine—Great Britain—History
I. Title II. Series
362.1′0941   RA418.3.G7
ISBN 0–333–39865–3

Series Standing Order

If you would like to receive future titles in this series as they are published, you can make use of our standing order facility. To place a standing order please contact your bookseller or, in case of difficulty, write to us at the address below with your name and address and the name of the series. Please state with which title you wish to begin your standing order. (If you live outside the United Kingdom we may not have the rights for your area, in which case we will forward your order to the publisher concerned.)

Customer Services Department, Macmillan Distribution Ltd
Houndmills, Basingstoke, Hampshire, RG21 2XS, England.

Editor's Preface

WHEN this series was established in 1968 the first editor, the late Professor M. W. Flinn, laid down three guiding principles. The books should be concerned with important fields of economic history; they should be surveys of the current state of scholarship rather than a vehicle for the specialist views of the authors; and, above all, they were to be introductions to their subject and not 'a set of pre-packaged conclusions'. These aims were admirably fulfilled by Professor Flinn and by his successor, Professor T. C. Smout, who took over the series in 1977. As it passes to its third editor and approaches its third decade, the principles remain the same.

Nevertheless, times change, even though principles do not. The series was launched when the study of economic history was burgeoning and new findings and fresh interpretations were threatening to overwhelm students – and sometimes their teachers. The series has expanded its scope, particularly in the area of social history – although the distinction between 'economic' and 'social' is sometimes hard to recognise and even more difficult to sustain. It has also extended geographically; its roots remain firmly British, but an increasing number of titles is concerned with the economic and social history of the wider world. However, some of the early titles can no longer claim to be introductions to the current state of scholarship; and the discipline as a whole lacks the heady growth of the 1960s and early 1970s. To overcome the first problem a number of new editions, or entirely new works, have been commissioned – some have already appeared. To deal with the second, the aim remains to publish up-to-date introductions to important areas of debate. If the series can demonstrate to students and their teachers the importance of the discipline of economic and social history and excite its further study, it will continue the task so ably begun by its first two editors.

L.A. CLARKSON

Editor

The Queen's University of Belfast

Introduction

THIS survey examines the social history of the impact of disease upon English people and of their responses to it, both lay and medical. Its chronology, roughly 1550–1860, spans early modern times and the first century of industrial society; this allows questions to be asked both about continuing traditions and about change (e.g. the effect of the Industrial Revolution upon the people's health).

It broaches some issues which are primarily demographic, by asking what part disease and medicine played in population changes. It touches upon economic history, by examining the changing wealth and market power of the medical profession. And it asks some questions best answered by the administrative or political historian (what role did the state play in promoting public health?). But it is not chiefly any of these – nor, above all, is it a reassessment of the roots of the welfare state or of the National Health Service [77]. Rather its main concern is with how people responded to sickness and to the threat of death – socially, religiously, medically. How relations changed between the people at large and the medical profession is central to that story.

In its organisation this pamphlet combines thematic and chronological approaches. The first chapter briefly sketches the 'biological ancien regime' as it affected English society between Tudor times and the onset of industrialisation. How severe were the threats which disease posed to population levels and social continuity? Did medicine offer people any real defences against disease? Chapter 2 then focuses upon the social presence of medicine in pre-industrial England. How was healing practised and who practised it? Was it largely the preserve of professional doctors, or did it lie in the hands of the people as well?

Chapter 3 explores from the inside this world of short lives and sudden death. What did it feel like to live in times when health and life itself were both so precarious? What did people think of doctors and the services they offered? How far did people try medical self-help? Or were they fatalistic, resigned to their fate or to the will of God? Seventeenth- and eighteenth-century attitudes are chiefly considered, but they still apply largely in the nineteenth century.

The fourth chapter then examines in greater detail the medical profession as it developed from the eighteenth century. Who were the doctors? What social place did they occupy? How many were there? What types of practitioners were there, ranging from the orthodox to the irregular and the out-and-out quack? How well did they meet the demand for medical services in an economy increasingly geared to 'consumerism', i.e. the provision of goods and services in return for cash payment?

If Chapter 4 examines doctors in their 'private' relations to their clients, the patients, Chapter 5 goes on to consider practitioners in their collective and public roles, particularly in the nineteenth century. How did the many distinct, and often competing, types of practitioner making up medicine as a whole relate to each other? How and why did medicine consolidate itself as a prestigious profession, rather than remaining just another 'white-collar' occupation like school-teaching or journalism? The answers to these questions are obviously bound up with the growing employment of medical men by the state in the nineteenth century as part of its new commitment to public health. This entry of medicine onto the public stage will be assessed.

In terms of saving 'endangered lives' [104], what did all this amount to? Could the rise of the medical profession, linked to a new 'scientific medicine', and the public health movement, with its 'sanitary science', do much to reduce morbidity and mortality? Were English people healthier in 1850 than in 1750, 1650 or 1550? Were they living longer? And if so, how far was it thanks to medicine? Such issues are tackled in Chapter 6. An important problem emerges: if medicine was still not very successful in preserving health and conquering disease even in the mid-Victorian era, how do we explain the growing presence and power of the medical profession in that society?

Fierce debates have raged between rival schools of historians as to how to interpret the march of medicine since Victorian times, culminating in the National Health Service, inaugurated in 1948. Doctors have generally stressed the part played by advances in medical science: scientific medicine has packed increasing curative power. Historians by contrast have stressed the importance of reform, humanitarianism and state intervention. By contrast, recent radical, feminist and Marxist scholars have offered more sombre revisionist interpretations: in their eyes, the rise of modern medicine is a story of professional aggrandisement, monopoly and profiteering, and of the use, or abuse, of medical power for 'social control'.

Certain prefigurations of these contesting viewpoints will emerge in this survey. But not many, for the interpretation of medicine's place in pre-industrial society has not been much debated. Research has remained fragmented. The aim, therefore, in the absence of a book-length survey on this subject, has been principally to draw together the threads of specialised publications.

Generalisations presented here will all too often rest upon flimsy evidence. Partly this is because vast areas still remain to be researched. Thus only one in-depth study has been written of how a hospital operated within an industrialising community [70], and only one full-length 'biography' of a lunatic asylum has been published [23]. The dangers of generalising from such single cases are obvious. But partly the problem is that the past is too often silent: vital evidence simply has not survived. Thus it is highly probable that large numbers of female healers ('wise women') possessed valuable medical skills in traditional society: indeed, feminists have claimed that 'witches' played an important medical role. Unfortunately, whereas a fair number of autobiographies and case-books survive, written by male practitioners, we lack equivalents from female healers. Their outlooks and practices must be deduced from second or third hand. Unequal survival of material and the biases of scholars mean that we know less about 'lay' medicine than about 'professional', less about 'irregular' than about 'official' therapies. That does not mean that the former were less important. Not least, the lower down the social scale we look, the less the information, and the less satisfactory it is. Moreover, despite the heroic efforts of historical demographers, all attempts to provide statistical profiles of life chances before the first census in 1801 are necessarily tentative [106].

This survey covers England, not Great Britain. It says nothing about Ireland and Wales, and very little about Scotland [34], or, indeed, the expanding empire. These regrettable gaps mirror the uneven state of current research. Here and there, however, a contrast with Continental Europe or America has been introduced [90] to highlight socially unique features of English medicine. Little is said either about epidemiology, or about the progress of medical science as such. For these McGrew [54] provides a useful reference work. For a longer time-span and a more international perspective, see [10], while for popular narratives of medicine and society see [94; 101; 102].

1 Disease, Death and Doctors in Tudor and Stuart England

Radical Puritans in the English Revolution (1642–60) wanted to transform the nation's institutions 'root and branch'. Not least amongst the evils they detested and aimed to change was the existing medical profession. Reformers such as William Dell thought that medicine had been perverted by the corrupt, privileged clique of physicians who controlled London's Royal College of Physicians, chartered in 1518, and thereby exercised power over other practitioners. This elite, bookishly trained in Greek medicine through a protracted university education, dogmatically upheld (certain reformers alleged) the exploded medical system associated with the authority of Galen and other 'Ancients'. By using the powers granted it by royal charter to regulate membership, and thereby to police London medical practice, the College oligarchy, bent on power and profit, was blocking the spread of newer, more progressive approaches to healing, in particular the Paracelsian, which was more popular and open, and favoured cheaper, simpler drug remedies [99]. Doctors, complained Lodowick Muggleton, were 'the greatest cheats in the world' [93, *17*].

In critics' eyes, the universities and medical colleges had combined to pervert English medicine, so that it provided unlimited but worthless treatment for the rich and all too little for the rest. Radicals proposed numerous schemes to reorganise it. They vowed to make medical education, knowledge and practice far more open, above all by replacing Latin with English. They proposed state-funded 'research centres' for the advancement of medical science along the lines advocated by Francis Bacon. And they advocated public provision of free or cheap medical facilities, including hospitals, for the sick poor, along lines which distantly anticipated the National Health Service [99].

The Puritans were right to think that medicine had little to be proud about. The shortcomings of Oxford and Cambridge in providing medical education were highlighted by the fact that most of the top English physicians had studied abroad, mainly in France and Italy. In any case, only a small percentage of medical practitioners had attended university, and these learned, gentlemanly physicians clustered in London, where the Court, City and Parliament provided the highest concentration of rich patients. Outside London, acdemically trained doctors formed a small minority; thus 5 out of 75 practitioners known to have operated in Norwich – then England's second largest city – between 1570 and 1590 had been to university [98]. Most practitioners had at best gained their skills as surgeons or apothecaries (roughly equal to today's dispensing chemists) by apprenticeship. They had no formal anatomical or scientific training.

Above all, critics denied that traditional medicine did much good. The prating, pompous physician, spouting Greek aphorisms, was an easy satirical target; and the experiences of the decimating waves of influenza and 'the sweat' in mid-Tudor times, or the dreadful epidemics which devastated the Stuart age – in particular, the successive outbreaks of plague, culminating in the carnage of 1665 – did nothing to enhance doctors' reputations [87]. It did not help, for instance, that most fellows of the College of Physicians fled London during the 1665 outbreak, or that the royal physicians made such a botch of the last illness of Charles II.

Worse still, medicine patently had no answers to the fatal diseases which time and again proved such scourges. The first half of the seventeenth century was a time of a marked deterioration in the climate, poor harvests, frequent dearth and chronic malnutrition caused by excessive pressure of population upon resources. Against this background, epidemics of typhus, scarlatina, measles, other fevers and, most terrifyingly, of bubonic plague, struck and struck again, checking the population rise which had been such a conspicuous feature of the Tudor century. In early Stuart England, life expectancy may have been under 35 years [15; 21]. Infants and children were particularly vulnerable. Of Samuel Pepys' ten brothers and sisters, only two survived into adulthood. Many factors combined to leave the population vulnerable: poverty, death, chronic fatigue, repeated pregnancies, insanitary and overcrowded living conditions. But in England – contrary to the experi-

14

ence of many parts of Europe – it was disease, rather than famine, which actually killed so many people [2].

And against such diseases, the healer's art proved a broken reed. The strengths and weaknesses of 'learned medicine' for those who could afford it were still those of the medicine of Antiquity, particularly that of Galen, on whose authority it leant so heavily. It set great store by the management of a healthy life through the regulation of diet, exercise and the pursuit of moderation. It also prided itself upon its clinical perceptiveness, bred of centuries of experience. But its powers for combating disease had advanced very little since the Ancients. The accent of its therapeutics lay on expelling toxic substances from the body – by purging, sweating, vomiting and the much favoured surgical technique of blood-letting – on restoring 'balance', and on strengthening the body's own regular constitution. To this end, a host of medicaments was used. Time-honoured simple herbal preparations had long been augmented by complex and often very expensive drugs, such as theriac, compounded of dozens of ingredients, many deriving from Arab medicine. Certain chemical and metallic medicines, such as antimony and mercury – pioneered by the sixteenth-century medical iconoclast, Paracelsus – were also being brought into the repertoire of drugs. Many of these preparations 'worked', in the sense that they brought about the predicted effect: they did indeed cause purging or vomiting. But very few of the recipes which physicians prescribed and apothecaries dispensed 'worked' in the larger way that, say, penicillin works, i.e. by destroying the micro-organisms which caused people to die from diphtheria, pneumonia, typhus and a huge range of infectious fevers.

It was basic science which would eventually enable late-nineteenth- and twentieth-century medicine to combat bacteria and sepsis. Seventeenth-century doctors lacked this. Neither had pharmacology proved very successful in coming up with 'wonder drugs' or even very effective pain-killers. Paracelsus had advocated mercury as a specific against syphilis, that new scourge introduced into England in the late fifteenth century – and that had proved reasonably effective, if highly unpleasant. Otherwise the drugs front was bleak. Even Jesuits' Bark (Peruvian Bark or quinine, a product of the cinchona tree), effective against fevers, and opium (powerful as a sedative and for bowel disorders), had made little inroad into England by the mid seventeenth century.

Surgery could offer little more. Surgeons performed a multitude of useful items of 'external medicine', dressing wounds, manipulating dislocations, lancing boils, pulling teeth and not least, letting blood, though in the days before the importance of scrupulous cleanliness was understood, even these routine treatments, performed with dirty hands and tainted instruments, might prove hazardous. Surgeons also set broken bones, all too common mishaps in a work-world in which almost all power was manpower, and in which travel by horse on rutted roads meant high casualty figures. Experience had taught, however, that all but the most simple breaks turned septic or gangrenous. Hence, faced with a compound fracture, surgeons would generally amputate (again hazardous, and a nightmare experience for the sufferer at a time before effective anaesthetics).

Unlike today's surgeon, however, his seventeenth-century forebear undertook little internal surgery. Malfunctions of the heart, liver, brain or stomach were treated not by the knife but by medicines and management. Brave people like Pepys would submit to the surgeon's knife for the common complaint of a bladder stone rather than endure lifelong excruciating pain. Pepys was one of the lucky ones who survived unscathed [72]. But major internal surgery was not feasible before the advent of anaesthetics and antiseptic procedures in the mid nineteenth century. A surgeon would very occasionally cut open a dying woman in labour to deliver a baby which could not be born naturally, but there is no record of a mother surviving a Caesarian operation in England till the close of the eighteenth century [24; 84]. In general, the only bodies surgeons were accustomed to cutting open were dead ones, for post mortems or anatomical instruction.

In other words, in early modern times, medicine was still losing the struggle against disease. Nowadays, when we fall sick, we expect medicine to cure or at least relieve us, and with good reason. Not so, three or four hundred years ago. This is not to say that people always despaired of the doctor and derided his physic. The medical profession was clearly in demand. Neither were all measures against disease hopeless. As Slack's study of plague has proved, energetic measures were commonly taken – more so in the seventeenth than in the sixteenth century – to halt the spread of the pestilence; travel and trade were restricted, families in which plague had struck were strictly quarantined within their own homes, domestic animals were destroyed, infected buildings were fumigated [86; 87]. Such measures might in a limited way be effective. The strict precautions taken by Thomas Wentworth, President of the Council of the North, in 1631 to protect York – he isolated the city and pulled down the squalid shanty-town suburbs outside the city walls where the poor lived – perhaps explain why that city escaped pestilence whereas others such as Bristol and Hull succumbed. Yet these were administrative and police measures rather than medical cures (in some ways anticipating the claim made by many nineteenth-century sanitary reformers that the politician could do more for public health than the physician).

Despite all these efforts, it remains clear that early modern medicine had no real answers to the epidemics which not uncommonly swept away a tenth of the inhabitants of a village within a year, or to diseases which killed off up to half the new-born babies, young infants and children under the age of five, not to mention so many women in child-bed, so many wage-earners and mothers in the prime of life. Thus vulnerable to attack, orthodox medicine had critics aplenty: alternative healers, satirists, fundamentalist preachers (who condemned it all as vanity: the cure of souls not of bodies was what counted) and those Puritan reformers with their blueprints of public medicine for all.

Despite all the criticism, almost nothing was achieved. The Puritan Revolution came and went without restructuring, redistributing or augmenting medical provision in England.

2   The Practice of Medicine in Early Modern England

WHEN people fell sick, what medical facilities were available for them in sixteenth- or seventeenth-century England [98]? The reasonably well-off might have access to three kinds of regular practitioner. At the top was the physician, whose job it was to diagnose the complaint, prescribe treatments and medicines (which the apothecary would then dispense), and provide attendance and advice. 'Physic' called itself a liberal profession, founded upon a university education. Physicians to the well-born and wealthy were expected to have a gentlemanly bearing to match that of their patients. The top physicians crowded into the capital, where fellows and licentiates of the Royal College of Physicians enjoyed a monopoly of practice [13]. Around 1600, London physicians numbered towards fifty, and the College jealously and zealously upheld its privileges through the courts. Outside the metropolis, physicians practised in smaller numbers in corporate towns and cathedral cities, where a better class of patients could be found. At least eleven physicians practised in Norwich between 1570 and 1590, six of them academically trained. Beyond that, the presence of university-educated physicians in country towns was haphazard, though many claimed to practise 'physic'.

Lower in status than the physician was the surgeon. His was a craft rather than a 'science', involving the 'hand' not the 'head'. His job (and occasionally, *hers*, for there were a few female surgeons) was to treat external complaints (skin conditions, boils, wounds, injuries, etc.), to set bones and perform simple operations. Because both were arts of the knife, surgery and barbering had, within the guild-system, long been yoked together, the Barber Surgeons Company of London dating from 1540 (the two did not go their own separate ways till 1745) [19]. The basic entry qualification for admission into the London Company, or into its equivalents in other corporate towns, was to serve a formal, indentured apprenticeship, generally for a period of seven years.

Somewhat parallel to the surgeon was the apothecary. Within the profession, the apothecary had low status because he kept shop and pursued 'trade'; his education was the 'mechanical' one of apprenticeship rather than the liberal one of the university. The apothecary was seen by the physician as his underling. The physician prescribed: the apothecary made up the prescription. Naturally much rivalry arose between the two branches; knowing more about drugs than physicians did, apothecaries attempted to prescribe on their own authority (humbler people were glad of this, since it cut out the physician's stiff fee). In London this led to friction and legal wrangling between the College of Physicians and the Worshipful Society of Apothecaries (founded in 1617 and legally subject to supervision from the College of Physicians) [10; 20]. Through the seventeenth century the College of Physicians generally managed to uphold its rights, though at the cost of losing public support. Outside London, however, such feuds were rare. They could flare up only where different grades of practitioner were separately organised or were treading on each other's toes. Neither really happened. In Norwich, for instance, surgeons and physicians were organised in the same guild [98], and in the countryside there was generally just a single practitioner in a particular area, who would turn his hand to all sorts of healing, no matter what his precise training or title. Certainly by the eighteenth century the name 'surgeon apothecary' was the commonest title given to the country or small-town practitioner (whether he had been trained and qualified in both or not), signalling the obvious need for the doctor to practise all aspects of medicine. In all but name, he had already become the 'general practitioner' [5; 52].

We do not as yet know how many regularly-trained practitioners were at work in Tudor or Stuart England. We can be sure that numbers steadily rose during the eighteenth and nineteenth centuries. The first national 'medical register', published in 1779 and 1783, lists about 3000 (the total must have been somewhat higher) [48]. We should not automatically project backwards from this and assume that doctors were in shorter supply in Tudor and Stuart times. Painstaking research by Webster and Pelling has uncovered impressive numbers of early practitioners. In London around 1600, some 50 physicians, 100 surgeons, 100 apothecaries and 250 additional 'irregulars' were practising, to say nothing of midwives and nurses. Provincial towns might be similarly well-stocked. The names of almost a hundred practitioners active in Norwich between 1550 and 1600 are known [98]. Rural areas, however, were prob-. ably much more poorly served. It might be indicative, for example, that the Revd Ralph Josselin, vicar of Earl's Colne in rural Essex, who kept an exceptionally full diary between the years 1643 and 1683, almost never called in a physician or a surgeon despite the endless stream of illnesses and accidents he and his family suffered [71].

Even where medical regulars were in short supply, there was never any shortage of other people experienced in caring for the sick. Such 'empirics' or 'irregulars' came in many guises. Some practised full-time, others occasionally; some for money, others out of charity; some were licensed, most were tolerated, a few were prosecuted. Amongst recognised practitioners were authorised midwives (all female). These required a licence from the local bishop which basically testified to the woman's good character. Morals and religious orthodoxy rather than medical skill were the criteria of fitness to attend births, because midwives so easily fell under suspicion of dabbling in abortion and conniving at the infanticide of bastard babies. How competent traditional midwives were is a matter of historical dispute. The male 'accoucheurs' – or obstetricians – who supplanted them in polite society during the eighteenth century depicted the old 'granny midwife' as ignorant and inept. Recent research has shown, however, that many mid-wives were literate and came from respectable families. They prob-ably managed normal deliveries well, though they may have lacked the expertise, practice and instruments needed to cope with excep-tionally difficult births [7; 24; 84].

Another type of medical practitioner who might have the legal protection of a licence was – paradoxically – the street-corner quack or 'empiric'. Mountebanks, mainly from France and Italy, could purchase royal privileges to practise just as 'empirics' (practitioners with no formal training) could patent their 'nostrums' and pro-prietary medicines. Ever pinched for money, Stuart monarchs were glad of the income derived from selling these rights, although the medical elite found it a scandal. In any case, the Stuarts had a stake of their own in irregular healing, since it was their practice to 'touch for the king's evil' (i.e. scrofula): in 1712 the young Samuel Johnson was to be one of the last people so 'touched' [8].

Thousands of other people made a living, or topped up their income, from medicine at this time. Grocers and pedlars sold drugs. Blacksmiths and farriers drew teeth and set bones, doubling in human and veterinary medicine. Itinerants toured the country, selling bottles of brightly coloured 'wonder cures' and moving on to the next town fast. Some were probably utter rogues like the mountebank in Ben Jonson's *Volpone*. Other travelling doctors possessed genuine skills in treating eye, teeth or ear complaints, thus performing a useful service in the days before business was brisk enough to support permanent, resident opticians or dentists in small country towns.

Far more people, however, practised healing without any view to reward, but out of motives of neighbourliness, paternalism, good housekeeping, religion or simple self-help. Every village had its 'nurses' and 'wise women' well versed in herb-lore and in secret brews and potions, their medicine perhaps merging into white or black magic. The gentry and clergy prided themselves upon their knowledge of physic, and treated their tenants, households and parishioners as a matter of piety, duty and sheer necessity. Their wives would also play 'lady bountiful' to the sick. As surviving manuscripts and printed recipe books show, possessing skills in home-made medicines formed as much a part of good housewifery for a lady as making her own soap, beer and preserves out of the produce of the kitchen garden, woods and hedgerows [71].

Some lay people went beyond this, and claimed a special gift of healing. For instance, the Irish gentleman, Valentine Greatrakes, discovered he could cure through laying on of hands. His fame spread, and he came to England, holding healing sessions even before Charles ii, to the sceptical consternation of physicians and scientists alike. One distinguishing feature of the 'free spirit' religious sects flourishing in the Civil War period was faith healing. George Fox, and other early Quakers, even expected to raise people from the dead.

Sometimes this 'lay' medicine was attacked by regular practitioners. But almost all was perfectly legal (only irregulars who brazenly trespassed upon the privileges of the London Colleges and Companies or the provincial guilds, found themselves indicted before the courts); and it filled a gap for those who could not afford regular practitioners, those who lived too far from them, and not least, for those who distrusted putting their lives in doctors' hands and who thought, by analogy with radical Protestantism, that every man should be his own physician.

Thus although professional doctors were fewer in Tudor and Stuart times than in later centuries, the presence of an abundance of popular healers meant that few who sought medical attention would have gone without. And that includes even the very poor. Physicians and quacks alike often made a point of treating some poor patients *gratis*, out of charity [64]. Moreover, institutional philanthropy helped a number of the sick poor. Certainly the Reformation under Henry viii and Edward vi had destroyed most charities designed to give refuge and medical care to the sick, the old and the infirm. In London, few institutions of medical consequence had survived the Reformation except St Thomas's Hospital, St Bartholomew's Hospital and Bethlem Hospital (popularly called Bedlam: England's only madhouse). By European standards, seventeenth-century England was exceptionally ill-endowed with hospitals or plague-houses, or with sister institutions such as orphanages. Yet local historical research is now revealing that more small alms-houses and hospices were being founded by charitable bequests than was once thought.

Moreover, within the framework of the Elizabethan Poor Law, modified at the Restoration, parish paternalism frequently involved no small outlay of ratepayers' money on the sick or infirm, out of a mixture of genuine neighbourliness and enlightened self-interest. The sick were commonly committed to the care of other poor parishioners paid to nurse them. Medicines, foods and funerals would be provided, and doctors' fees reimbursed for treating the poor. In the eighteenth century it became common for a parish to contract with a particular general practitioner to treat its paupers for a fixed sum per year. Sometimes the amounts laid out on individuals appear surprisingly generous. It was not unknown to pay to send a sick person to a spa or to London for treatment, doubtless hoping that such outlays would in the long run prove cheaper than the cost of permanent parish relief. Pauper hospitals were a rarity under the Old Poor Law (Bristol pioneered the pauper hospital, as it pioneered the workhouse); but in the days before friendly societies, charity and Poor Law relief combined to offer at least some medical attention to the lower orders [65; 92].

3 Experiences and Actions: Countering Illness in the Seventeenth and Eighteenth Centuries

PEOPLE of all age groups, occupations and social classes in early modern England knew they trod the pilgrim's progress of life in the shadow of sickness, disability and death. As they walked through the churchyard on Sunday or listened to the preacher, adults saw close around them massive evidence of death: tombstones or tablets commemorating their grandparents, one or both parents, brothers and sisters who had died in infancy, and not least their own children. Youngsters would grow up wearing the clothes of dead siblings. It was common for the newest born to be given the name of a dead brother or sister. Christianity itself hinged upon the great mystery of death; funerals were celebrated infinitely more lavishly than marriages or baptisms, and somewhat later, new secular cultural forms also gave great prominence to mortality, not least newspaper obituary columns [31].

In such a society illness and death were bound to loom large in people's minds. This is certainly confirmed if we read the age's sermons and works of religious comfort, and above all if we survey the fragmentary remains of individual opinions: commonplace books, journals, letters and diaries [71]. Such sources are of course socially unrepresentative – they record the thoughts of a tiny minority of exceptional, literate people in a society in which a majority were illiterate. At least before the eighteenth century, our first-hand evidence from women is scanty, and such documents give almost no insight into the minds of children. But letters and diaries do tell us much. Their writers regularly witness deaths in the community. Illness is a constant theme – of the diarist himself, his family and friends. What is more, such documents give glimpses (at least) of a wider 'sickness culture', showing beliefs about the meaning of life and death, about the causes and purposes of sickness, about its prevention and cure, the relations between body and soul, flesh and spirit, mind and matter. For the early modern mind, the condition of the body, registering the ups and downs of health and sickness, meshed with wider ideas of identity and destiny, of social, moral and spiritual well-being.

Furthermore the personal preoccupation with sickness – found in letter writers and diarists such as Samuel Pepys and the Puritan Richard Baxter – mirrored larger concerns. Remedies against sickness, omens about death, consolations for sufferers: these loomed large in a popular culture passed down orally, almost literally with one's mother's milk, but they were also intoned from the pulpit, read in the Bible and other religious works, and even picked up from the printed health-care manuals which first started appearing in Tudor times and had become extremely widely read by the nineteenth century [71; 98]. We cannot assume that people believed all that doctors told them about medicine, or all that preachers thundered about the corruption of the flesh. Contemporary diaries record just how often the writers ignored their doctors' advice. They did not always follow the recommendations they heard or read (how many people nowadays avidly read health-care columns and continue to smoke or over-eat!). But there was clearly some congruence between 'public opinion' and private experiences: and this allows us, however tentatively, to piece together the fragments of the 'sickness culture' of the centuries before the Industrial Revolution and before the emergence of modern, scientific medicine.

To do this, it may be helpful to contrast it with assumptions widespread today. Nowadays for most people, health is the normal expectation, sickness an annoying and temporary interruption to a lengthy span of healthy activity – maybe seventy years – whose termination seems sufficiently remote that it can safely be put out of mind. Thus disease is seen as an exceptional intrusion. Falling ill can generally be explained (in line with a popular image of Pasteurian bacteriology) as the result of the invasion of one's body by 'pathogens' from outside, colloquially called 'germs' or 'bugs'. Thus we 'catch' flu. It is then the job of the doctor, aided by science and technology, to kill this invader, with the aid of miracle drugs, especially antibiotics, and to relieve suffering with 'pain-killers'. Alternatively, other kinds of illness are seen as due to some 'breakdown' in the body's mechanism, the failure of a part such as a hip joint or the heart; generally in hospital, while

24

the sufferer is unconscious under anaesthetics, this can be mended or the part can even be 'replaced'. The patient wakes up 'better' [35].

This outline picture can be called the 'medical model' of physical illness. Disease is regarded as an alien entity. It strikes from outside for no particular reason. It afflicts our 'body' – which is not quite the same as our 'selves'. And we trust the doctor to repair our body, rather as we expect the mechanic to mend our car. Overall, illness has no particular meaning and the doctor is the active agent, the hero even, in its conquest.

Little of this would have rung true to Tudor or Stuart sufferers, or even to most Victorians. Then, illness was typically seen not as a random accident striking from outside, but as a deeply significant life-event, integral to the sufferer's whole being, spiritual, moral and physical. This was partly because of contemporary assumptions about what caused illness. Both the explanations of the doctors, reflecting the best classical theories, and the outlooks of lay 'common sense', regarded health as a measure of the proper workings of the individual constitution, and sickness of its malfunctioning. In maintaining good health, one needed to ensure proper diet, exercise, evacuations, adequate sleep and the like. It was important to live in a healthy environment, regulate one's passions, and be moderate and temperate in habit.

More particularly, the different forces vital for life had to be kept in equilibrium. The body must not become too hot or too cold, too wet or too dry, and this in turn depended upon maintaining the right balance between the key fluids (technically called 'humours') which made the body work – for example, the blood. Sickness was the result when the body balance was disturbed. If the system grew too hot and dry, this was expressed in fever; if too cool and wet, then it developed a 'cold'. If too little blood were produced, the body lacked nourishment and languished. If an excess of blood were generated (for example by eating too much red meat) one's blood would boil or it would rush to the head; 'hot blooded' people were liable to apoplexy (a stroke). Thus sickness was largely seen as personal and 'internal'. Such 'distempers' could be treated by restoring the lost equilibrium; hence 'cooling' herbal medicines, blood-lettings or even cold baths would be good for fevers, plenty of rich food and red meat would cure 'thin blood'. But better still, careful attention to all aspects of 'regimen' (or lifestyle) would prevent 'disease' (literally 'dis-ease') in the first place [71].

Thus bouts of sickness, from minor discomforts to dangerous fevers and seizures, were typically seen as integral to the individual's constitution and personality. This implied the opposite of today's 'doctor dependence': your life was not in his hands but in your own. Such views made good sense at a time when curative medicine was little advanced (as explained above in Chapter 1) and the physician's healing power extremely limited. It also harmonised with an often expressed faith in the 'healing power of nature' (*vis medicatrix naturae*), a common-sense recognition of the self-limiting nature of most ailments. One way that people in traditional society coped with the fact that doctors were not miracle-workers was to view their own health as ultimately their personal responsibility. As will be seen below, this belief had important consequences when it came to deciding what to do when one fell sick.

But if, anatomically and physiologically speaking, keeping well was in theory chiefly a matter of leading a balanced, regular, moderate life, why did people so often fall sick and die? There were several plausible overall explanations. For one thing, far too many people lived in bad environments or pursued unhealthy occupations which were bound to lead to disease. Ever since the Greeks it had been common knowledge that overcrowded, airless quarters of towns were hotbeds of epidemics, or that people who lived in marshy areas frequently got 'ague' (malaria). The blame lay (it was believed) with poisonous gases (miasmas) exhaled from the earth. Only vigorous motion, free currents of air and fast-flowing water, would break these up and dispel them. Likewise, it was well known that potters got lung diseases, or that lead-workers were liable to paralysis: such diseases just came with the job [100].

Second, it was widely believed that disease might be the result of *maleficium* (spells cast by witches) or of satanic or demonic possession. Keith Thomas has shown how belief in witchcraft, magic and demonology gradually declined during the seventeenth century – precisely why is less clear – and it seems that attributing sickness and death to evil spirits, and countering these by magical remedies, increasingly became confined to the lower orders, to the countryside and to oral culture. Nevertheless survivals of medical magic, such as passing a child with whooping cough under a donkey, still flourished in the nineteenth century, and it long remained acceptable to attribute certain forms of disease to the Devil. Even in the eighteenth century, John Wesley, the founder of Methodism (and in many ways a pioneer of new scientific medical therapies, such as the use of electric shocks) regarded insanity as typically caused by diabolical possession [3; 93].

Third, and extremely importantly, the fallen condition of mankind was blamed for the ubiquity of sickness, suffering and the empire of the Grim Reaper. Through their original sin, Adam and Eve had brought disease and death into the world as punishments for disobedience. The Bible warned that women would bring forth children in pain, as a consequence of the sins of the flesh. Seventeenth-century Protestantism believed the end was at hand, the world was old and decaying fast, and the proliferation of plagues, epidemics, disasters, dearth, famine and wars was to be seen as the mark of the imminent Dissolution. Disease could thus be a perpetual *memento mori*, and death itself a release from this vale of tears [31].

Such views could make general sense of the empire of disease and death. They did not, however, satisfactorily explain the personal dilemma: *why did it happen to me?* Today, because most diseases are just passing interludes, we rarely endow them with special meanings. In the seventeenth century, when life was precarious and death commonly struck in the prime of life, and the salvation of the immortal soul was paramount, each illness episode had to be scrutinised for its deeper meanings. And so, as the thoughts of contemporary diarists show, sickness was interpreted as full of moral, spiritual and religious messages. Often it seemed the workings of natural justice. The sins of the parents would be visited upon their children. Thus adulterers would contract venereal infections, and the idle would be punished with melancholy. Even the worldly Pepys saw some of his illnesses as retribution for his sexual misdeeds.

But above all, sickness was regarded as the finger of Providence. God used illness for a multitude of higher purposes. It could often be an affliction against the ungodly, like the Old Testament plagues hurled against the Egyptians. Thus bubonic plague was widely interpreted by the pious as a punishment, as a reminder of Divine Wrath, and as a warning to the wicked to mend their ways. But there were positive sides to Providence too. When the Puritan

27

Richard Baxter fell sick and thus escaped involvement in some disagreeable business, he thought the hand of God had spared him; it was a kind of Divine medical certificate. For the Revd Ralph Josselin, the fact that the pain of bee stings could be soothed by applying honey was further proof of divine Providence, in supplying ready remedies for doubtless well-deserved afflictions. In any case, physical pain in turn served as God's reminders about far worse spiritual torments. For Josselin, a bee sting girded him against the far more dangerous sting of sin [71].

Thus sickness became one of many ways God revealed His will to man. Belief that disease had divine meanings did not, however, supersede the idea that it also had natural causes to be treated medically (compare Cromwell's instruction to his troops to 'trust in God and keep your powder dry'). Few people thought that medicine and the Divine will were at odds, though some Scottish Calvinists later judged it impious to inoculate against smallpox (if it was God's will that one contracted smallpox, it was sacrilege to prevent it). Muslims took few precautions to avoid plague, seeing it as a blessed mark of divine favour. But such religious fatalism was rare in seventeenth-century England. Worries about how to square Providence with medicine seem more common in the nineteenth century, with the emergence of religious sects such as the Christian Scientists.

The medical culture of pre-industrial England was thus centred upon the individual, and God's purposes for him, more than upon disease or the might of medicine. This had important implications for what people did in the teeth of illness. For one thing, diaries and letters show that people paid great attention to the causes of sickness and took steps to avoid it. The cautious expended much effort in choosing their diet in keeping warm (a particular concern of Pepys), and in taking exercise. Those who could afford it visited spas such as Bath, bathed and drank the waters [80; 94]. Many diarists routinely dosed themselves with tonics, gave themselves purges and emetics, and called in the local barber-surgeon to let blood, as steps in a self-administered regime of health. In the eighteenth and nineteenth centuries, many further ways of toughening the constitution, strengthening the fibres and cleansing the system gained followers, including gymnastics, cold-water bathing, vegetarianism and teetotalism. Putting prevention before cure, and Nature before the doctors, became the trade mark of the theories of the lay-dominated medical fringe in the nineteenth century [8; 42].

Moreover, autobiographical evidence shows that when people fell sick, it was important for them to form their own diagnosis. Symptoms are rarely recorded without an accompanying stab at an explanation. When Pepys went down with stomach pains and fever early in 1663, he puzzled himself for a cause, deciding it was 'some disorder given the blood: but by what I know not, unless it be by my late great Quantitys of Dantzicke-girkins that I have eaten'. In the face of such danger, finding an explanation was reassuring. It quelled anxiety. But it also helped sufferers to make their next important decision: whether to summon professional help or not. Nowadays many people automatically go to the doctor as soon as they feel sick. But no one in early modern society – except of course certain hypochondriacs – routinely sent for the doctor when they felt ill, even badly ill. No one thought that professionals had a monopoly of medical sagacity. Nobody regarded it as offensive to their physician to try self-diagnosis and self-dosing first, or expected to incur his wrath by so doing.

So people pondered their symptoms and attempted their own diagnosis. Very often, they would then administer medical self-help. Well-stocked homes had kitchen-physic: bottles of home-brewed or shop-bought purges, vomits, pain-killers, cordials, febrifuges (medicines to reduce fever) and the like. At least by the mid eighteenth century it was common for families to stock up with patent and proprietary medicines such as Dr James' Powders, the Georgian equivalent of aspirin. By the nineteenth century products still familiar today, such as Eno's Fruit Salts and Beecham's Pills, were appearing. One could also buy ready-made medicine chests. The aid of friends, family, 'wise women' or the squire might also be sought. Contemporary letters abound with recipes and treatments recommended in response to news of ailments. Recipe-books and health-care manuals bulge with home remedies for all kinds of disorders from corns to cancer [8; 57].

Of course, self-medication is universal. But the sick a couple of centuries ago were probably much more self-reliant and less doctor-dependent than today. That is not surprising. Doctors then had no magic bags of tricks. Educated lay-people might reasonably feel – unlike nowadays – that they could understand medicine on a par with the professional. Moreover, there was no range of drugs

29

which could be obtained only from the doctor, on prescription. Till well into the nineteenth century, all drugs – even dangerous ones such as opium – and poisons as well could be bought over the counter [8].

But what happened if the sick person decided to call the doctor? Much depended upon social class. Today's general practitioner commands professional authority, and is backed by science, diagnostic technology, laboratory tests, specialists, consultants and the prestige of the hospital [85]. Great things are expected of him. That was far from the case three centuries ago. Practitioners were often of lower social status than their gentry clients; they were expected to show due deference. Not least, patients of rank clearly expected doctors to fall in with their own auto-diagnoses and favourite treatments. In the eighteenth century Samuel Johnson – a man who respected doctors, though he was a particularly cantankerous patient – sometimes gave orders to his doctors. On one occasion, against his physician's advice, he insisted that his surgeon bled him. (Johnson had faith in heroic remedies, believing that 'pop-gun batteries' did no good; a fact which suggests that the vogue for vile-tasting brews crammed with disgusting ingredients may have been to satisfy sick people's desire to feel that medicines were really acting.) As late as the beginning of the nineteenth century Dr Thomas Percival, in his pioneering book on medical ethics, advised physicians to fall in with the desires of their wealthy patients to have particular medicines prescribed, while of course denying any such indulgence could be allowed to poor charity patients in hospitals [43].

In modern doctor-patient relations, the doctor is in the driving seat, so much so that radical critics of the profession, such as Ivan Illich, have reiterated George Bernard Shaw's gibe that medicine is 'a conspiracy against the layman' [41]. This description hardly applies three centuries ago. In the seventeenth century the profession as a whole commanded little corporate power, and few individual physicians attained great celebrity or wealth. The diaries of eighteenth-century patients show that they often disregarded their physician's advice, and dismissed bossy practitioners. They felt no compunction about shopping around for second and third opinions, and made free use of quack and unorthodox remedies as well, following a try-anything mentality which gave no automatic privilege to regular medicine [71].

30

In the long run, the collective prestige of doctors would rise, the patient would be more firmly fixed 'under the doctor', and consumers would lose some of their say. These developments will be traced in Chapters 4 and 5. But that rise was slow. Scepticism about physic long continued. Popular proverbs endorsed this distrust ('one doctor makes work for another'), and echoed the Biblical: 'physician, heal thyself'. Physicians were pilloried in novels as 'Dr Slop', 'Dr Smelfungus', or collectively in Hogarth's engraving as the 'Company of Undertakers'. The public would have agreed with the kind of resignation expressed by Elizabeth Montagu in 1739:

> I have swallowed the weight of an Apothecary in medicine, and what I am better for it, except more patient and less credulous, I know not. I have learnt to bear my infirmities and not to trust to the skill of physicians for curing them. I endeavour to drink deeply of philosophy, and to be wise when I cannot be merry, easy when I cannot be glad, content with what cannot be mended, and patient where there can be no redress. The mighty can do no more, and the wise seldom do as much. [72]

It is perhaps then revealing, that at least up to the end of the seventeenth century, physicians were rarely present at life's two greatest crises, birth and death. Traditional child-birth was attended by midwives and 'gossips' (i.e. friends and neighbours) but not (except in emergencies) by medical practitioners [7]. Similarly with death-beds. The tactful doctor would tell his patients that they were dying, to give them time to put their affairs in order, and recognising that there was no more for him to do, would retire, leaving the last hours to the family and perhaps a clergyman. In the medical *ancien regime*, sufferers and doctors could co-exist without undue tension, because the limits of medicine's powers were clear to all.

4   Medicine in the Market Economy of the Georgian Century

THIS survey has argued so far that medicine led a chequered existence in Tudor and Stuart England. Although the nation boasted a few great medical scientists – of whom William Harvey, discoverer of the circulation of the blood, and the astute clinician, Thomas Sydenham, are the most eminent – the professional elite had more enemies than friends, and was indicted for being monopolistic and self-serving without offering correspondingly successful medical care. Neither the College of Physicians nor the Company of Surgeons did much for medical education or research (the Royal Society, chartered in 1662, was somewhat more productive, staging the first experimental blood transfusions). Seventeenth-century attempts by Puritan reformers and by advocates of the new chemical drugs to change the structure of organised medical practice or to establish new theories and therapies met with resistance.

It would be easy to paint a picture of medicine in eighteenth-century England meandering along in the same course, still unreformed, only yet more oligarchic: the increasing exclusiveness of the Colleges mirroring and being sheltered by the Walpolean political system of 'Old Corruption'. Indeed, that is precisely how nineteenth-century reformers – spearheaded by the journal, the *Lancet*, founded by the surgeon and democrat, Thomas Wakley– viewed things in their crusades against the medical establishment. Historians have commonly endorsed their reading, seeing the eighteenth century as an era of medical stagnation, at last swept aside by a new broom in the 'age of reform', which put an end to privilege and nepotism, and opened up the careers to talent.

Indeed, there is much to be said for this view. By no criterion did the College of Physicians or the Company of Surgeons improve the standards of English medicine under the Hanoverians. The

College suffered some reverses around the turn of the eighteenth century, falling out of royal favour, and (after the House of Lords' judgment in the Rose Case, 1704) losing its monopoly right to prescribe medicines in London [16]. Henceforth, the Lords ruled, apothecaries might also prescribe, provided that they charged only for their medicines, not for their advice. (One dubious effect of this judgment was that it gave apothecaries every incentive to palm off ever increasing quantities of medicines on their patients; many apothecaries just ignored it, however.)

Following this defeat, the College grew introverted. It exercised its police powers to prosecute unlicensed practitioners far less (for which dereliction of duty later reformers roundly abused it), and turned into an exclusive club, reserved for gentleman physicians. The College successfully resisted all calls to open its fellowship to London physicians at large. Its statutes normally reserved admission into its fellowship – where all the power and prestige lay – to graduates of Oxford and Cambridge and members of the Church of England. Certainly by the second half of the eighteenth century many of London's best physicians were Dissenters by religion and had been trained either at Leiden in Holland or at Edinburgh University, which by then boasted perhaps the top medical school in the world. Eminent physicians such as the Scot, William Hunter, and the Quakers, John Fothergill and John Coakley Lettsom, intensely resented being consigned to remaining mere 'licenciates' of the College: non-voting members, or, in other words, second-class citizens. Their campaigns to open up the College met with diehard resistance [13; 96].

The Surgeons' Company likewise made scant contribution to medical advance. The formal separation in 1745 of the Surgeons from the Barbers did at least establish that surgery was a craft in itself, a cut above mere hairdressing: but the divorce accidentally spelt a backward step as well, since the new premises occupied by the Surgeons long lacked a dissecting theatre. (One of the *raisons d'être* for the Surgeons' Company lay in its privilege of conducting public dissections of executed criminals – important in an age when anatomical knowledge was increasingly seen as crucial to every surgeon's training.) [19]

If the London corporation did little for medical education, English universities achieved hardly more. The output of medical graduates from Oxford and Cambridge during the eighteenth century

33

sank far below the levels reached in the previous century. Most medical professors were nonentities, who rarely lectured, and Oxford and Cambridge missed out on one of the key advances made at Leiden and Edinburgh, the integration of lectures with clinical instruction in an adjoining hospital. Overall, Georgian England failed to provide medical training adequate to its needs. By the end of the eighteenth century, top London physicians, the cream of provincial physicians, and the leading hospital and army and navy surgeons – an increasingly important branch of the profession – were getting their medical education elsewhere, above all in Edinburgh, which pioneered *university* education for surgeons and not just for physicians [74].

Last and not least in this diagnosis of Georgian decay, is the fact that medicine remained formally straitjacketed in its traditional, three-tiered, hierarchical structure (physicians, surgeons and apothecaries, in descending order), their relations soured by jealousy and rivalry. This legal and institutional division of labour was increasingly archaic and did not conform to the facts of medical practice. After all, from 1704 London apothecaries had the right to practise physic, though not to be paid for it. And in the provinces the great majority of regular medical men, whatever their training or licence, operated neither as physicians, surgeons nor apothecaries, but as all three, as general practitioners [5; 52].

The failure of this medical superstructure to reform itself to meet the times meant that Georgian doctors remained easy targets of satirical attack, being presented as living fossils, wedded to their dead learning. Yet this is only part of the picture, and not the most important part. Overall, medical care grew rapidly in the eighteenth century – in quantity and probably also in quality – and the standing of medical practitioners rose alongside. This was the product of various trends [33].

For one thing, most ranks in Georgian society were enjoying a century of increasing prosperity. England came to boast ever-expanding middling classes of merchants, tradesmen, shop-keepers, clerks, farmers, skilled craftsmen and the like, with money to spare even after the necessities of life had been supplied. Such families sought to ape their betters, to spend more upon services, commodities and consumer items. Amongst the many outlays increasingly recorded in their account books – alongside money spent on library subscriptions, hairdressers, music lessons and suchlike –

were payments to medical practitioners. Men whose mothers had relied upon the village midwife now booked the accoucheur to deliver their wives' babies; women whose grandmothers had mixed family brews now bought proprietary medicines for their ailments or called the surgeon-apothecary. Medicine expanded as part of the general growth of the service sector in a thriving consumer economy.

At the same time, lay initiatives led to new medical institutions being set up. In their political outlooks, men influenced by the Enlightenment were keen to promote secular welfare, the health as well as the wealth of nations. They also set great store by humanitarianism and philanthropy. Many traditional types of charity, however, such as religious good works and educational foundations, only exacerbated animosities in a society already deeply politically and religiously divided. Hence the new hope was that medical charities, by contrast, would prove a social balm, not an irritant. Partly for these reasons, the Georgian century witnessed quite unprecedented private giving for medical good causes – in particular, the founding of hospitals and, later, of dispensaries. Such institutions were typically meant for the poor (though not for Poor Law paupers), who would receive care without charge, thus, it was hoped, confirming ties of deference, gratitude and paternalism.

London benefited earliest from the wave of new foundations. To the metropolis's two ancient hospitals, St Thomas's and St Bartholomew's, a further five were added in quick succession between 1720 and 1750: the Westminster (1720), Guy's (1724), St George's (1733), the London (1740) and the Middlesex (1745) [9; 14; 22; 75]. All these were general hospitals. They set off a wave of similar institutions in the provinces, where, until then, no genuinely 'medical' hospitals had existed at all. The Edinburgh Royal Infirmary was set up in 1729, followed by Winchester and Bristol (1736–7), York (1740), Exeter (1741), Bath (1742), Northampton (1743) and some twenty others. By the end of the eighteenth century all sizable English towns had a hospital [105]. The old corporate towns and cathedral cities got them first, the newer manufacturing centres such as Birmingham and Manchester later.

Augmenting these general foundations, Georgian philanthropy also pumped money into more specialist institutions for the sick, particularly in London, but elsewhere too. Charitable donations

35

led to St Luke's Hospital being opened in London in 1751: the only big lunatic asylum in the kingdom apart from Bethlem. Unlike 'Bedlam', widely criticised for its barbarity and lack of therapy, St Luke's was launched to an optimistic and progressive fanfare, its physician, William Battie, asserting that, if treated with humanity, lunacy was no less curable than any other disease. By 1800, other great towns, such as Manchester, Liverpool and York, had their own public lunatic asylums, philanthropically supported [45].

As well as lunatics, sufferers from venereal disease also became objects for charity, perhaps indicating the waning of the traditional religious judgment that such diseases were punishment for vice, and its replacement by the Enlightenment view that humanity demanded the relief of suffering. London's 'Lock Hospital' for venereal cases opened in 1746. It was paralleled by another new charitable foundation, the Magdalen Hospital for Penitent Prostitutes (1759). This was less a medical hospital than a refuge, in which prostitutes who wished to 'go straight' could stay, learn a trade, and prepare for a new life. Another important type of new voluntary hospital was the 'lying-in' hospital. In London, the earliest of these maternity hospitals were the British (1749), the City (1750), the General (1752) and the Westminster (1765). Maternity hospitals met several major needs. Not least, they guaranteed a few days' bed-rest to poor women living in overcrowded tenements and beset by the constant demands of large families. Also, because some did not insist that the mother-to-be should be married, they enabled unmarried mothers – commonly servant girls – to deliver their illegitimate offspring with no questions asked. Many of these babies then ended up in the Foundling Hospital, opened in 1741 as London's first major orphanage (unwanted children could be deposited there, anonymously; they would be brought up, educated and taught a trade) [53; 64].

Lying-in hospitals served a further function. From the start they were centres of tuition and practice for trainee midwives and for the newer male accoucheurs or man-midwives (today's obstetricians). All these desirable functions were offset by one grave drawback. In the days before sepsis was understood and the importance of scrupulous cleanliness recognised, maternity hospitals readily became deathtraps. Mother and baby mortality was higher in these hospitals than with home delivery [95].

One further important movement of medical charity gathered

pace from the 1770s: the dispensary movement. Hospitals aimed to provide treatment, nourishing food and bed-rest. By 1800, London's hospitals alone were handling between 20,000 and 30,000 patients a year. But they restricted themselves to fairly minor complaints which would respond to treatment, excluded infectious fever victims (no one wanted fever epidemics raging uncontrollably through the hospital), and in any case, could treat only a fraction of the sick. Hence it became important to augment hospital facilities. One device was the fever hospital, designed only for infectious cases. London's fever hospital (tactfully known as the House of Recovery) was opened in 1801. If it could do little for typhus, dysentery cases, etc., it could at least help halt the spread of such infections by isolating their victims. But the key device was the dispensary. The first London dispensary was set up in 1773. By 1800, sixteen dispensaries existed in London, treating up to 50,000 cases a year, and many in the provinces besides. Dispensaries mainly provided outpatient services, supplying advice and free medicine to the sick poor for whom there was no room in hospitals or whose complaints were unsuitable for hospitalisation. More important, perhaps, the dispensary system involved domiciliary visits by eminent physicians into the homes of the poor. This first-hand experience of how the other half lived fired the reforming zeal of progressive doctors for improved housing, better sanitation and health education for the people [51].

These initiatives transformed the English medical landscape. The voluntary hospital movement did not amount to the comprehensive, state-funded medical system which some seventeenth-century Puritans had envisaged (that had to wait until 1948). Neither did it spark any major breakthroughs in medical science or therapeutic powers: it is one thing to provide VD hospitals or mental hospitals, another to cure their victims. Such foundations did, however, signal a new recognition on behalf of opinion-makers that the health of the people mattered. Piety and humanity demanded compassion for the sick; utility taught that neglecting disease ran counter to enlightened self-interest: for diseases readily spread from the poor to the better off, and sick and disabled labourers made inefficient employees. In the light of these moral considerations, it is not surprising that the initiative for institutional advances generally sprang from laymen, not doctors. Thomas Guy, whose money set up Guy's hospital, was a London printer; Thomas

Coram, inspirer of the Foundling Hospital, was an old sea-dog: Alured Clarke, who laid the blueprints for many provincial voluntary hospitals, was a clergyman. Subscriptions for such foundations generally came from nobles and gentlemen, rich merchants, clergy and civic worthies: and as generous donations carried votes on the governing boards, the management of these hospitals and charities largely remained in the hands of the laity, with physicians taking a back seat.

Of course, the hospital movement greatly benefited the medical profession as well. Every hospital had one or more honorary appointments for physicians and surgeons. They would give their services free (or for a nominal honorarium) as an act of public generosity. However, the honour and publicity accruing from hospital appointments proved career 'leg-ups' for ambitious practitioners, who could expect, through the hospital, to hobnob with the best society amongst the governors, and thereby gain powerful patrons and wealthy private patients. Hospital appointments, especially in London, could prove more directly lucrative as well: hospital staff, especially surgeons, took apprentices who would walk the wards, and learn the craft while acting as the surgeon's assistant. It was the ideal apprenticeship, and the surgeon could command good fees. Moreover, especially after about 1750, London hospital doctors began to deliver lecture courses on subjects such as anatomy, materia medica, surgery and practical physic, on hospital premises. Popular courses drew scores of students, whose fees would entitle them not just to attend lectures but to have open access to the hospital wards. Thus the habit grew up of 'walking the wards': generally, the students were in tow to the physician or surgeon as he did his rounds, explaining cases as he went from patient to patient: sometimes they inspected on their own [38].

Thus hospital expansion gave rise to teaching in the hospitals. Even if this was not as formal or systematic as the medical education provided from the 1820s by 'teaching hospitals' proper (such as University College Hospital, or the Charing Cross) it at least represented a great educational leap forward, by bringing together theoretical and practical instruction. If English universities did nothing for improving medical education in the eighteenth century, voluntary hospitals made up for some of their defects [7; 61; 74].

The hospital movement thus provided benefits for the medical profession. But ultimately it began as, and remained, a lay initiative.

It showed that the polite and the propertied recognised that if wealth was to enjoy security it must wear a human face; they saw that the wealth of nations depended upon the productive toil of the respectable labouring classes; common sense taught it was prudent to keep such people fit to work.

It was also a response to the fact that in a free-market industrialising society – using more complex and dangerous machinery and more toxic chemicals – working people were bound to be crippled by occupational diseases and industrial accidents. A few employers, such as the potter Josiah Wedgwood, set up private sickness insurance schemes, through which the workforce, in return for a compulsory deduction from their wages, became entitled to medical treatment and sick pay. But most capitalists and employers of domestic servants chose to make contributions to hospital charities, which would entitle them to admission tickets for their own employees. The setting up of specialised charities also points to growing awareness of the hazards of industrialisation. The Royal Humane Society (founded in 1773) aimed to teach techniques of artificial resuscitation to save those rescued from drowning. With ports, rivers and canals playing such key roles in economic expansion, many fell victim to the hazards of water (it was also said that the proverbially suicidal English made a habit of throwing themselves off bridges in despair). Other societies were set up to provide free surgical appliances to those engaged in heavy labouring jobs whose working life was threatened by ruptures. Such institutions continued to function and expand throughout the nineteenth century, indeed up to the founding of the NHS [100].

Society thus recognised it could benefit from expanding medical demand, both private and public. Doctors in response were ready and able to profit from the new opportunities. At the head of the profession, the medical elite grew more opulent, more fashionable, more prestigious than its Stuart equivalent. This had little to do with any new medical skills. It was more a matter of top physicians proving themselves cultured, civilised, and urbane – the kind of men High Society, and not least Society ladies, felt they could trust and admit to their circles. Physicians such as Hunter, Lettsom, William Heberden and Matthew Baillie won faithful clienteles, widespread plaudits and social acceptance through clinical acumen, courtesy and good breeding which avoided both old-fashioned pedantry and uncouthness [7]. Other physicians made their social mark as cultural lions. Both Richard Mead and Sir Hans Sloane dabbled in science and built up fabulous collections of antiquities, books and *objets d'art* (Sloane's collection, bequeathed to the nation, became the nucleus of the British Museum). The surgeon William Cheselden was a friend of Alexander Pope and designed a bridge over the Thames at Putney. Others won *entrée* by shining as men of letters: Samuel Garth, Richard Blackmore, Mark Akenside and Erasmus Darwin were probably equally famous as poets and as physicians (Tobias Smollett and Oliver Goldsmith were doctors whose literary career outstripped their medical).

For top physicians such as these, incomes soared. William Cheselden could reputedly charge £500 for a lithotomy operation (a good 'piece' rate, since his forte was to extract a bladder stone in less than five minutes): £500 was the annual income of many a country squire. Lettsom, Mead, Hunter and Baillie probably topped £10,000 a year, an income unknown in earlier centuries and equivalent to the rent roll of a lesser lord [7].

But good times spread right down the profession. Recent research by Loudon has shown that the fees which small-town apothecaries and country surgeons could command steadily rose during the eighteenth century [52; 36]. Business also became brisker. A provincial physician such as Erasmus Darwin could make over £1000 a year in the latter part of the century, country general practitioners could net £500, and the cream of the provincial apothecaries, such as William Broderip of Bristol, had incomes running into thousands. Such men bought themselves country houses and rode around in carriages whereas their predecessors had gone horseback. Doubtless they worked hard for their rewards (Erasmus Darwin reckoned he travelled 10,000 miles a year); and doubtless only a few did so well, though all the signs point to a substantial general drift upwards of medical incomes in a century in which, before the 1780s, there was little inflation. Overall, Georgian affluence – helped by the secular temper of the age, where the claims of the body counted more than those of the soul – spelt good times for doctors [36; 52].

They were, moreover, helped by the emergence of profitable sidelines. As already noted, hospital posts became available, offering prestige and admission into the higher circles of town life, and the promise of future profit. Other country practitioners topped up their income by engaging in 'contract' Poor Law practice. The developing medical speciality of man-midwifery provided further opportunities. A specialist London man-midwife could charge fees running into hundreds of guineas to deliver titled ladies who found it more fashionable and perhaps safer to have a well-trained, genteel male practitioner rather than the traditional midwife. Outside London, obstetrics was increasingly practised by surgeon-apothecaries. They shrewdly perceived that the doctor who successfully delivered a baby won lasting gratitude and the mother and child as patients for life. Obstetrics smoothed the way for the rise of the family doctor [85].

Another lucrative new sideline could be smallpox inoculation. Inoculation (deliberately infecting healthy people with a mild dose of smallpox, to provide future immunity against what often proved a fatal, or at least, a badly disfiguring disease) had been introduced into England in the 1720s by Lady Mary Wortley Montagu (a lay person, not a doctor), who had seen it as a folk practice in Turkey. The English medical profession proved quite receptive – more than the French – and the practice was given good publicity by the willingness of the royal family to have their children inoculated. From mid century, inoculation became common in the countryside (it worked best in small communities, where mass inoculation was feasible). Often it was performed by general surgeons, who could charge a guinea a jab. But certain practitioners chose to specialise as inoculators. The most successful were the Sutton family. In twenty years they claimed to have performed 300,000 inoculations, bringing an annual income of several thousand pounds. Even luckier was Thomas Dimsdale. A country physician who had made a speciality of inoculation, he was invited in 1768 to St Petersburg by Catherine the Great to inoculate herself and her son. His reward was £10,000, plus £2000 expenses and an annuity of £500 [58; 76].

In fact, various new routes to fame and wealth were opening for the medics. Some, like John Pringle (who ended up as President of the Royal Society) chose to make a name for themselves in army or navy medicine (in an age of warfare and imperialism, military medicine offered splendid career prospects for enterprising young doctors) [46; 50]. Others began to specialise. As earlier described, traditional medical theory, following the Greeks, saw sickness as a symptomatic disorder of the whole system rather than as specific to a particular organ, and so it tended to stigmatise as a quack the man who claimed to treat a single condition or organ in isolation (that was the fate even of eye-doctors who operated for cataract). But circumstances gradually changed that. In particular, Edinburgh University was turning out increasing numbers of highly skilled graduates, trained both in physic and in surgery, whose prospects of becoming a fashionable London bedside physician were thwarted by the restrictive practices of the College of Physicians. In the late eighteenth century and beyond, many looked to specialisation as their route up the career ladder. Some, as already mentioned, became specialist man-midwives. Eye, nose, throat and cancer specialists followed.

Others turned their main energies to medical instruction. From early Georgian times a handful of practitioners were giving lecture courses for students in London and, by the close of the century, teaching was standardly being offered in the hospitals. But on top of these, several enterprising practitioners founded their own private anatomy schools in London, the most famous being set up by the Scot, William Hunter, in Great Windmill Street in 1765. Proprietors gave extensive medical instruction to all who could pay the fee of a few guineas – Hunter's course ran to 112 two-hour sessions. But, more important, they catered for the practical side of the art, by providing plenty of demonstrations and specimens preserved in bottles and showcases; and, a key innovation, they gave students first-hand anatomical experience by providing corpses for dissection. For this, entrepreneurs such as Hunter had to enter into shady and illegal dealings with London's underworld of body snatchers ('resurrection men'). Private anatomy schools offered the best medical education in London until they were superseded by the teaching hospitals from the 1830s [7; 18].

A further expanding field of medical specialisation which opened new careers and spelt fame and fortune was the treatment of lunacy. Before 1700 the insane were rarely locked up in madhouses. England's only public madhouse, Bethlem Hospital, housed only about a hundred lunatics. As noted above, a number of public asylums were set up during the eighteenth century, funded by philanthropic donations. But the main growth came in the private sector. There the 'trade in lunacy' grew up, based upon the private madhouse. Enterprising doctors and keepers would set up premises for confining the insane, charging stiff fees paid by their friends and family. In some, the insane were merely kept in safe custody; in the more ambitious asylums, early versions of psychiatric therapy were also given. Private madhouses were profitable business propositions in the free market economy. They were utterly unregulated by law until 1774 (and thereafter, though licensed, were still subject to little supervision). The worst were riddled with abuses; patients were mistreated, and sane people were sometimes shut up in them just to keep them out of the way.

Some of these private asylums, however, were reputable institutions run by high-minded doctors anxious to specialise in insanity and develop psychiatric expertise. A typical Edinburgh medical graduate, Dr Thomas Arnold, set up an asylum in Leicester and published a pioneering two-volume psychiatric textbook. He won the recommendation of James Boswell, who had a disturbed brother who had to be locked up, and who was no stranger to depression himself. More spectacular, however, was the success of the Revd Dr Francis Willis, a Church of England clergyman who had turned to medicine and set up his own high-class private asylum at Gretford in Lincolnshire. When George III became delirious in 1788, and his general physicians failed to restore him, Willis was called in. His brusqueness with the King (he put him in a straitjacket) and his unorthodox treatments (which included 'fixing' his patients with his 'eye') caused raised eyebrows, but George recovered (if only temporarily), Willis took the credit, and was voted a £1000 p.a. pension by Parliament.

Insanity was to remain a promising field for the enterprising doctor. Unlike in Catholic countries where religious orders bore the brunt of care, in England the field was left free for the individual madhouse proprietor, who did not even need to be medically qualified. Not until 1845 was it compulsory for local authorities to build asylums on the rates. Even after then, most mad people from 'respectable' families were confined in the comparative seclusion of private asylums. Thus insanity proved yet another condition which doctors steadily made their territory during the eighteenth and nineteenth centuries, a further opportunity for medical practitioners to thrive in England's flourishing and largely *laissez-faire* society [45; 67].

We might thus assume that regular medicine grew during the Georgian and early Victorian eras at the expense of lay and irregular practice. Certainly midwives felt they were being elbowed out by the ambitious new accoucheur. The 'wise woman' receded into the shadows. The Victorian antiquarians who patiently collected medical folk-lore believed they were witnessing a dying tradition [3].

Yet many fields of irregular medicine were actually growing alongside the rise of regular physic, surgery and the apothecaries' trade. In other words, the total national appetite for medicine was rising fast, and the public which, in a free market, ultimately voted with its pocket, was eager to sample whatever systems, therapies and drugs were on offer. After all, regular medicine had no corner on effectiveness: and although plague had mercifully quit England after 1666, the eighteenth and nineteenth centuries proved times when fever epidemics had lost none of their power to kill, and in which certain 'new' diseases, such as rickets, consumption (tuberculosis) and typhoid associated with foul urban living conditions grew more common. With regard to medicine, the law basically adopted the free market maxim of *caveat emptor* ('let the buyer beware'). In these conditions irregulars, quacks and patent medicine vendors seized the opportunities a hungry market offered. With good reason, the eighteenth century has been called 'the golden age of quackery'.

To speak of quackery is not automatically to impeach the motives of empirics (i.e. unqualified practitioners) and nostrum-mongers, nor to pass judgment on their cures as necessarily ineffective. Many of the most famous (or infamous) Georgian quacks, such as James Graham, advocate of mud-bathing, vegetarianism and sexual rejuvenation, were fanatics, all too fervent believers in their own powers. Likewise many proprietary remedies were remarkably similar to those physicians prescribed, sharing the same active ingredients such as opium (as a pain-killer) and antimony (which induced sweating to reduce fever). In this case it could make good economic sense to prefer ready-made nostrums simply because they were cheaper. In fact, the best approach to understanding quackery is to see it as the entrepreneurial sector of medicine. Here few practitioners were regularly trained, unorthodox methods were to the fore (such as the use of electric shock therapy), and practitioners drummed up custom by advertising and spectacular publicity, rather than by cultivating a settled general practice by patronage, or word of mouth recommendation. They made their profits out of selling commodities (above all, nostrums) rather than from receiving fees for advice, expertise and bedside attendance [8].

The traditional Italian-style charlatan, gaudily dressed and aided by a stooge and a monkey, setting up his stage on the street corner, gathering a crowd by his patter, drawing a few teeth, giving out free bottles of julep, selling a few dozen more, and riding out of town, was by no means extinct in Georgian England. Such figures could still cut a dash and make a fortune; even in the late nineteenth century witness 'Sequah', an 'American' mountebank who created a national sensation by performing 'Red Indian' rituals and vending 'Indian' remedies [82]. Most mountebanks, however, were probably small-timers, like the man who had a circuit in rural Sussex in the mid eighteenth century (as Thomas Turner chauvinistically noted in his diary, *he* had seen through the fellow, though his wife was taken in).

But some made big money. Joanna Stephens hawked a remedy which promised to dissolve bladder stones without surgery. Eventually Parliament raised a £5000 subscription to buy the recipe from her. Joshua Ward made a fortune out of his 'pill and drop' nostrum, effective for all diseases. In the eighteenth century Samuel Solomon, William Brodum and numerous others, and in the nineteenth, James Morrison, Thomas Holloway and Thomas Beecham, all got rich out of proprietary medicines. The art was to offer to meet needs which regular medicine failed to supply. Thus patent medicines promised to cure otherwise fatal diseases such as TB, or to restore lost youth and vigour, or to treat conditions such as venereal disease about which patients might be embarrassed to consult their regular physicians. For instance, Solomon's 'Balm of Gilead' claimed to cure the alleged ill-effects of masturbation, while 'Hooper's Female Pills' were a barely disguised abortifacient.

Many leading entrepreneurs of the Industrial Revolution, such as Josiah Wedgwood, owed their success to exploiting consumer psychology and dextrously manipulating publicity and advertising. Similar arts were perfected by the leading lights of irregular medicine. Large promises, attractive packaging, seductive names, free gifts, special offers, money-back-if-not-satisfied guarantees, were the common coin of these pioneer products of the pharmaceutical industry. Above all, nostrum-mongers went in for saturation advertising – in the streets, and then endlessly in the newspapers, London and provincial, which became an ubiquitous feature of Georgian life. Newspaper agents also undertook to distribute drugs, so that country readers often found access to 'mail order' patent medicines easier than to regular doctors.

In these ways, eighteenth- and nineteenth-century medical opportunists cashed in on the self-diagnosing, self-help medical traditions deeply ingrained amongst the laity, while pandering to 'consumerist' desires for miracle cures and something new. Habits of self-dosing with 'over-the-counter' medicines were built up. The Victorian lower classes and their children swallowed gallons of laudanum, an opium mixture which eased pain and stupefied infants. The 'stop smoking fast' promises of today's small ads columns and the millions of bottles of useless cough syrups taken even now, are the legacy of the transformation of medicine into a commodity in the first 'consumer revolution'.

The development of a market-oriented, mass-sales medicine did not necessarily amount to 'fringe' medicine, if by that we mean medicine radically at odds with orthodoxy (e.g. homeopathy), advanced by opponents of the dominant medical elite [42]. Indeed, the top 'quacks' of Georgian England are more noteworthy for their desire for acceptance in fashionable society than for being champions of the common people against the Establishment. Many quacks, such as Joshua Ward, hobnobbed in High Society and with top doctors. A little string-pulling ensured that his 'pill and drop' became standard navy issue. For their part, too, regular doctors were not averse to profiting from nostrum-mongering. Dr James' Fever Powders were the property of a bona fide Oxford MD, respectable medical author, and friend of Samuel Johnson.

By the nineteenth century, things had changed somewhat. Both religious dissenters and political radicals increasingly rejected the values of the titled, the rich and the fashionable. Instead, individualism, liberty, purity and self-help came to express the ideals of self-improvement amongst the artisans and labouring men of the industrialising Midlands and North. Such people commonly wanted little to do with orthodox medicine or with the commercial nostrums they identified with Mammon. Instead they embraced a new medical sectarianism which went hand-in-hand with religious nonconformity and political radicalism. For some – mainly the petty bourgeoisie – homeopathy had an appeal. Its hostility to medical profiteering and its stress on the need for absolutely pure drugs struck chords with many. More widespread in appeal were various kinds of 'medical botany' (herbalism), including the Thomsonian or Coffinite movements, introduced from America. Herbal remedies, taken straight from nature and often compounded by the sufferers themselves, excluded professional exploitation and adulteration, and were thus the very essence of self-help. Jesse Boot, the founder of Boots Pure Drug Company, had his roots in medical botany, setting up in pharmaceuticals because he was dissatisfied with the impurities of the drugs commonly available [8; 12; 42].

This chapter has traced how broad perceptions of health needs changed, and were met, in an expanding capitalist society undergoing rapid industrial change. Affluence and secularisation diverted more resources into health care, and medicine increasingly took the form of a commodity. Like so many other occupations, medicine profited in these sunshine years, increasing in numbers and creating new niches. It became a more lucrative profession, and doctors were to occupy a more prestigious place in society; in certain manufacturing towns, like Manchester, they readily became civic luminaries [70]. Certain historians have argued that this growing medical presence amounted to 'medicalisation', whereby medicine claimed a say over increasing sectors of life [41]. But to regard English developments in these terms before quite late in the nineteenth century obscures more than it clarifies. For despite individual prosperity, regular medicine continued to exercise little *collective* public power, and to enjoy hardly any state backing. When Queen Victoria came to the throne, doctors were still largely beholden to the consumers, and the public was showing itself notoriously fickle in its choice of what kinds of medicine to prefer [44].

5 The Medical Profession and the State in the Nineteenth Century

IN 1823 the surgeon and democrat Thomas Wakley founded a radical medical journal, the *Lancet*. Wakley, the son of a Devonshire farmer, was a tough, aggressive radical who fought in boxing booths in his youth, once walked from Devon to London, and adopted the style of a bruiser in his editorials. Indeed, early readers of the *Lancet* might be pardoned for getting the impression that English medicine was rotten with turpitude and ineptitude. Wakley shot withering blasts at all the medical corporations, accusing them of neglecting their duties even as they abused their powers. London hospitals were nests of nepotism, one consequence of which was that the public suffered neglect, mistreatment and hamfisted surgery. Institutions purporting to protect the public in fact damaged its health. No wonder, argued Wakley, people patronised the sharks and swindlers whose careers as quacks ought to have been cut short by decisive Collegiate action. In the midst of all this corruption, only the honest surgeon-apothecary, i.e. the emergent general practitioner, upheld the standards of true medicine; and for his pains, he could hardly make a decent living [89].

We must take Wakley's wailings with a pinch of salt. A man of passion and prejudice, he habitually dipped his pen in bile. The early nineteenth century did indeed see great dissatisfaction, but that stemmed perhaps less from the feeling that the profession had reached rock bottom, than from a determination to secure better times ahead. Medicine was growing militant.

Wakley certainly got one element of his diagnosis spot on, however. He grasped how the different branches of medicine were at loggerheads (he himself was not averse to exploiting their divisions for tactical advantage). Central to his account of medicine's toils and troubles was the view that it would never enjoy its proper place and powers in society (which he believed should be large) while it remained fragmented into the antagonistic and obsolescent branches of physic, surgery and pharmacy, each headed by a self-perpetuating cabal which failed to represent the real interests of the bulk of its practitioners. Until the profession was reorganised, the sick could not be protected, fraudulent practitioners silenced, or the public served.

A farsighted parliamentary statesman could possibly have seized the nettle in 1800, 1820 or 1840, and restructured the profession from tip to toe. He would have received few thanks for his pains, and no politician reckoned it was his business – let alone to his advantage – to clean out the profession's Augean stables on its behalf. In the late eighteenth and early nineteenth centuries, parliamentary bills aimed to alter the regulation of medicine were rarely passed, and most of those that did were the work of MPs favourable to the wishes of the College of Physicians. Such was the Apothecaries Act of 1815.

This Act was the outcome of years of reformist agitation by provincial general practitioners, who claimed their livelihoods were being undermined by unfair competition from 'mere' druggists, and who complained that their interests were not protected by any of the London corporations. The Act itself specified that, in future, the normal qualification for practice as an apothecary should be possession of a licence issued by the Society of Apothecaries (the LSA), which involved an apprenticeship, taking stipulated courses, some hospital experience, and passing examinations. This represented a minor victory for general practitioners, since it established a clear legal boundary between the qualified apothecary and lowlier medical men treading on their tails, such as retail druggists [8; 39].

But on the wider issues, as Holloway has recently argued, it spelt a major set-back for the general practitioner, since nothing was done to regulate unqualified druggists (or indeed other quacks and empirics) or to give general practitioners, who constituted perhaps 90 per cent of all medical regulars, a governing body of their own [39].

The aftermath of the 1815 Apothecaries Act was recrimination rather than reconciliation. The divisions within the profession remained. London physicians and surgeons, securely in the saddle, were deaf to the arguments that in a transformed nation, whose population almost doubled from 6 million in 1760 to 11.3 million in 1820, new standards of medical education and skill required a restructuring of the profession. Further waves of reformist agitation rose in the 1820s and 1830s, including a campaign by rank-and-file surgeons against the self-perpetuating oligarchy running the College of Surgeons. Ordinary members of the College (MRCSs) had no vote in choosing its Council, which co-opted itself.

In the 1830s, in an atmosphere dominated by Parliamentary Reform and by the advent of cholera in 1831–32 (which only underlined the ineffectiveness of medicine), the British Medical Association was founded as a ginger group for GPs who aimed to open up the medical corporations democratically to all their members. But still the medical old guard carried sufficient clout in government circles to maintain the *status quo* [69; 97].

The reconstitution of the medical profession did not come until the 1850s. Again the internal pressure came from below. By the mid nineteenth century, the medical profession was, numerically speaking, utterly dominated by non-metropolitan general practitioners. There may formerly have been some sense in keeping them as a subordinate element of the profession, back in the days when the typical country surgeon was an old sawbones and the apothecary kept shop, and neither knew more medicine than an apprenticeship had taught. But that situation was long past. Many country practitioners now had a top-class medical degree, from Edinburgh, Glasgow, or in an increasing trickle, from the new London University. Those lacking a degree were generally now both Licentiates of the Society of Apothecaries (LSA) and Members of the Royal College of Surgeons (MRCS). Many now held responsible public office, as Poor Law doctors, as physicians to public lunatic asylums, or as surgeons to public hospitals. The disfranchisement of such men from their own professional bodies was becoming a scandal apparent both to alert leaders of the profession and to politicians.

For the fear was that unless regular medicine had reform imposed upon it by Parliament – it showed no sign of reforming itself – it would forfeit public confidence and lose ground to the other brands of medicine, commercial medicine such as druggists offered, fringe medicine and the medical sects, eventually suffering the fate of the medical regulars in the USA where, without legislative protection, orthodox medicine seemed to be losing to the sects in the battle for public favour [90].

The Medical Act of 1858 (and several less important subsequent pieces of legislation) proved an ingenious compromise, placating the reformers, protecting the profession, and ensuring that in the resultant readjustment of territorial boundaries, none of the regular profession came out as losers. To satisfy the Colleges of Physicians and of Surgeons, the tripartite division of English medicine was not abolished: the Colleges themselves survived unscathed. To satisfy general practitioners, however, these distinctions became for practical purposes meaningless. In future one single public register of all legally recognised practitioners would be promulgated, under the official authorisation of a General Medical Council (GMC). All would appear equally on it, from the plushest Harley Street consultant down to the humblest village LSA. The significance of the register lay of course in those it excluded. For all ranks of regular practitioners now appeared together as 'insiders', lined up against all the 'outsiders' – the unqualified homeopaths, medical botanists, quacks, bone-setters and the like, who were automatically constituted, by exclusion, into the 'fringe'. Parliament had achieved what the doctors never could; it had – symbolically at least – united the much-divided medical profession, by defining them over and against a common Other, not to say enemy [69; 97].

Moreover the Medical Act had teeth (though no very strong bite). Thenceforth it became a legal offence for those not on the medical register to represent themselves as medical practitioners (an offence akin to false pretences). To the chagrin of GPs however, the practice of healing by non-registered doctors was not made illegal. Parliament knew that any such ban would have been extraordinarily unpopular with the public and anyway utterly impossible to enforce. Practitioners not on the register, however, were disqualified from holding public medical office. Since doctors were increasingly gaining full or part-time paid public employment as Medical Officers of Health, Poor Law hospital doctors, forensic experts in the courts, asylum superintendents and so forth, this was a privilege worth having.

This public unification of the divided profession found institutional expression. The Colleges of Physicians and Surgeons remained, as did the Society of Apothecaries; but they were little more than ghosts of past glories. Henceforth two bodies would dominate within the modernised profession. On the one hand, the

51

British Medical Association (BMA) grew out of its rebellious youth as the GPs ginger group, and settled down to become the conservative voice of the profession. On the other, the General Medical Council (GMC) became the parliamentarily sanctioned official watchdog of medicine (though its members mainly came from within the profession). Its fundamental function was guardianship of the Register. The GMC would add names to the Register. More crucially, it would be the body which struck names off, for offences such as gross professional misconduct (this rarely happened). Through the GMC, the state ratified medicine's claims to be an autonomous, self-governing ethical profession.

The constitutional reorganisation of the 1850s has proved durable; this was partly because it mainly registered changes which the profession had already undergone. For, long before the 1858 Act ended the paper wars between physicians, surgeons and apothecaries, new professional regroupings had taken shape. London's elite physicians and surgeons had ceased to require the armour which Collegiate privileges provided. They had established themselves in new, secure and well-upholstered positions of eminence and authority. They had increasingly associated themselves with hospital medicine: prestigious not because of its patients, but because of the opportunities it provided for eminence in teaching, for gathering pupils, for making a scientific name, for exercising patronage, and for winning public recognition. The distinction of a practice in Harley Street, combined with a consultancy at a leading London hospital, with patients recommended by one's former pupils for whom one had found good practices in choice areas: these ensured that medicine continued hierarchical even after the old hierarchy was effectively dissolved [69; 73].

For the GP in Rochdale or Rotherham, however, the professional recognition – the semi-closed shop – offered by the mid-Victorian legislation amounted to little. He was a member of an ancient, learned, liberal profession and had probably invested far more time, energy and expense in his training than his father or grandfather. But his prospects depended almost wholly upon the market forces of supply and demand. Things worked out nicely for some. A senior practitioner in a county town, serving as honorary physician to the local voluntary hospital, might feel fortunate both in income and in status. But such were in a minority. For most GPs the Victorian age blew chill winds. Much of the problem was that the profession was growing overstocked for comfort. There were all too few genteel career openings for the Victorian middle classes who felt a cut above trade. Medicine fitted the credentials – but fitted them all too well. By mid century, Edinburgh, Glasgow, Oxbridge and London University were between them turning out hundreds of medical graduates a year. This number increased with the rise of provincial university medical schools later in the century. Without plenty of pull and capital to buy themselves into an established practice, such graduates were faced by the prospects of lean years of desultory practice in a provincial town, waiting for senior rivals to die off, or exploitation as a junior partner, in which the elder would treat his underling as a dogsbody and would pocket most of the fees. Dr Arthur Conan Doyle, a young GP in Southsea, took to writing detective stories because he had so few patients.

Reform-minded general practitioners had hoped that raising the admission requirements for the profession, forming a register and penalising unregistered practice would do the trick. But it did not. The only way GPs' financial prospects could be guaranteed to rise would have been through curbing entry into the medical schools, and pruning the graduate lists. But such 'restrictive practices' would have smacked too much of old Collegiate oligarchy or new trade unionism.

One need not shed too many tears over the living standards of Victorian GPs. On the other hand, it is not clear that most fared better than their forebears, the Georgian surgeon-apothecaries (to that extent, to speak of the *rise* of the GP, though true in one respect, hides an irony: to many it seemed more like a decline). Few came to a competent living (and all that that entailed, including the ability to marry respectably and start a family) before they were about forty. Most remained appallingly overworked, on call at all hours, fifty-two weeks a year. They had to be endlessly civil to snobbish affluent patients, willing to bear with slow payers and bad debts. Most ended up, willy-nilly, treating scores of the sick poor who never paid at all. And rivals were always at their heels [52; 66].

Particularly in the early stages of a career, practitioners often had to engage in practice which was arduous, distasteful and barely remunerative. Many young GPs became Poor Law doctors or workhouse medical officers, under the terms of the New Poor Law

53

(1834): agreeing to meet the medical needs of a 'union' of parishes at least guaranteed an income of a couple of hundred pounds a year. On the other hand, the elected Boards of Guardians were hard taskmasters, ever with an eye to saving ratepayers' money. Poor Law doctors found themselves saddled with gargantuan work loads. In 1836 Mr Wagstaffe of St Mary's, Lambeth, claimed to have seen 6000 cases of illness, made 20,000 visits, and sent 10,000 mixtures, 12,000 powders and 30,000 pills – all on a salary of £105 a year [88]. Many received far less.

Another expedient increasingly common during the century was to become a practitioner to the multitude of lay-run friendly societies and benefit clubs which provided medical attention and drugs to working men, generally in return for contributions of a penny (1d.) a week. Once again, the assured income was an attractive prospect. But such a position generally meant a galling lack of autonomy. Above all, the doctor had to please his patients, otherwise a rival would appear at the end of the year, make a lower tender, and supplant him. When patients complained about their treatment, friendly society doctors were always liable to be hauled over the coals by the lay committee. Patient power and client control were, from the point of view of doctors, an unconscionable time a-dying [32].

So making a successful career involved a thorny path for the conscientious general practitioner of mid-Victorian England. He was a vulnerable individual in a highly competitive, buyers' market, in which it was not uncommon for doctors to undercut each other or to poach patients. Moreover his medicine was still not much more effective than that possessed by his seventeenth-century counterparts: he would still be performing operations on the kitchen table or watching helplessly as patients in the prime of life succumbed to TB or babies died of summer diarrhoea. Hence he had to work hard to keep the confidence of disgruntled patients through being ever-ready to visit, generous with his time, and full of words of comfort: the classic bedside manner [85]. For an outsider the prospects of rising up the profession to become a top consultant were negligible: such men still largely came from a self-selecting elite.

In these circumstances it is hardly surprising that when Lloyd George introduced his National Insurance scheme in 1911 (whereby the state guaranteed medical treatment to contributing working men, through 'panels' of doctors who would be paid an annual capitation fee by the state), even though the BMA huffed and puffed, fearing doctors would forfeit their independence, the majority of practitioners joined the scheme, glad to have an assured income. This was repeated after the Second World War with the setting up of the National Health Service. The BMA, the possibly unrepresentative mouthpiece of the GPs, was hostile: it feared that NHS doctors would be reduced to the standing of post office clerks. The situation seemed far different to many hard-up practitioners, plagued by prickly patients and the spectre of bad debts. For them the prospect of an annual fee per patient, paid by the state, was a blessed release from insecurity. The great mass of general practitioners have never had it so good as under the NHS [29; 91].

The nineteenth century produced a paradox. For the fortunes of rank-and-file practitioners languished at precisely the time when the state at long last recognised the crucial importance of medicine and public health to the nation's well-being. Throughout the century, a succession of scandals, revelations and reports uncovered appalling health risks, failures in the public provision of elementary utilities such as water and waste disposal, and mismanagement of medical services: many of these the consequence of the staggering increase of slum housing, industrial pollution and occupational disease caused by rocketing population and unprecedented industrialisation [83; 103; 104]. The House of Commons Committees in 1807 and 1815 discovered barbarities in both public and private madhouses; the reports of the Poor Law Commissioners in the 1830s presented a welter of evidence proving that England's towns were death-traps for lack of adequate pure water, sanitation and sewage-disposal. Factory inspectors' reports showed how the workplace was a prime scene of disease, injury and accident. Successive visitations of cholera (the new plague) in 1831–2, 1848–9, 1854 and 1861, sparked urgent investigations of how filth, squalor and urban overcrowding provided perfect breeding-grounds for disease. Between them, Florence Nightingale and *The Times* correspondent, William Russell, revealed gross hospital mismanagement in the Crimean War [88].

Awareness of terrible health hazards and medical shortcomings was nothing new. Back in the late eighteenth century, the investigator and humanitarian John Howard had published two important works exposing the unhygienic conditions typical of English hospitals and jails. Medical contemporaries of Howard, such as Lettsom, explained how slums, overcrowding, urban filth and ignorance combined to create conditions ripe for lethal fever epidemics. The point is that such revelations provoked almost no parliamentary response in the eighteenth century. No Act of Parliament was passed instigating a general clean-up of prisons or inaugurating the removal of nuisances or slum clearance (in the nineteenth century, by contrast, airy new thoroughfares, such as Charing Cross Road and Shaftesbury Avenue, would be bulldozed through the most pestiferous rookeries, courts and alleys). This is not to say that the Georgians were indifferent to welfare. Rather action was left to local bodies such as vestries and parishes and – an important new development – to semi-private, semi-public bodies of 'commissioners', who would undertake responsibility for street cleaning, refuse-disposal, lighting and so forth, in return for the power, secured by private Act of Parliament, to levy a rate. From the late eighteenth century, such commissioners did good work in making most towns more habitable. They could not cope, however, with the sheer scale of the health risks of the nineteenth-century conurbation.

For a variety of motives – necessity was one, the zeal of the Benthamite and Evangelical lobbies another – the nineteenth-century state gradually adopted a more interventionist role. The revelation of scandals increasingly led to public response, however delayed and inadequate. Outcry over the evils of madhouses, for example, produced legislation in 1808 and 1845 setting up a nation-wide system of public lunatic asylums, and Acts of 1828 and 1844 establishing the Lunacy Commissioners whose job was to inspect madhouses and root out abuses [45]. Florence Nightingale's campaign led to a major reorganisation of military medical services and then of the nursing profession in general.

This is not the place to retell the story of the growth of public health services. These, particularly in the wake of the New Poor Law of 1834, whose board of commissioners was led by the indefatigable and dogmatic sanitarian, Edwin Chadwick, did much to alert the public to the unhealthiness of towns [29; 30]. Chadwick saw the solution in centralised powers to investigate the dangers caused by contaminated water, fetid cesspits, blocked drains, overcrowded churchyards and the like, to prosecute, and to legislate for improvements [27; 49; 107].

But two new trends should be mentioned. First, an infrastructure – however piecemeal – of medical or quasi-medical functionaries and of institutions was created from the 1830s, whose task was to safeguard the public health. Here it was crucially important that the New Poor Law (1834), which made the workhouse the statutory device for controlling England's growing army of paupers, also set up alongside the workhouse the Poor Law infirmary. The diseases of the indigent (increasingly regarded as menacing the entire nation) were now too dangerous to be left to neighbourly self-help, private charity or *ad hoc* parish relief. Once set up, Poor Law medical services expanded to meet the new needs which their own existence revealed and created. For example, fever and isolation hospitals were often added, and non-paupers, suffering from contagious diseases, were commonly removed to Poor Law infirmaries. In effect an NHS for the poor was being created a century before it was set up for the rest of society; though Poor Law medicine was characteristically cheeseparing, harsh and authoritarian, and was feared almost as much as the workhouse itself [1; 37].

Another crucial aspect of the creation of this infrastructure was the appointment of local Medical Officers of Health, made possible by the Medical Act of 1848 and compulsory by an Act of 1872. The first appointment was made by Liverpool. John Simon (later Sir John) was then appointed MOH for the City of London in 1848 [47]: others followed. A series of Nuisance Removal Acts (1855, 1860, 1863) gave MOsH powers to eliminate health threats from the environment (garbage tips, food adulteration, slaughterhouses, poisonous effluents and fumes and such like). Once set up, their powers grew, both to investigate and to prosecute. Georgian England had developed no equivalent of the 'medical police' bureaucracies common in Continental absolutist states. From the mid nineteenth century, however, England at last had its 'medical policemen' [29; 107].

Alongside this permanent infrastructure went new public attitudes, above all the idea, fitfully but increasingly apparent, that the interests of public health overrode sacred liberties of the person and of property. Reflecting on cholera, *The Times* pronounced in 1848 that it would rather take its chance with death than be bullied

57

into health [25; 59; 68]. Such individualist, *laissez-faire* views gradually lost favour and were overtaken by events. In the 1840s, Parliament empowered the Board of Health in a series of statutes to act on such issues as polluted water supplies, contrary to the rights of the private water companies. It marked a major extension of central powers. In a similar way, legislation of 1853 eroded the liberty of the person and invaded the sanctuary of the family by making smallpox vaccination compulsory [47]. This was drastic action indeed, given that a sizable minority of the population was, or became, violently opposed to vaccination, on grounds of science, religion and liberty. Slightly later, the Contagious Diseases Act (1867) continued the same trends. In an attempt to contain venereal disease in the British armed forces, Parliament gave magistrates powers in stated garrison towns and ports to detain any woman suspected of being a prostitute, submit her to medical examination and, if found diseased, subject her to compulsory medical treatment. This Act seemed to threaten individual liberty so dramatically, that it brought about an unlikely alliance of protests from old-style libertarians and new feminists.

By the time he came to write his eleventh annual report to the Privy Council in 1868, Sir John Simon could boast of the magnitude of the state's role:

> It has interfered between parent and child, not only in imposing limitation on industrial uses of children, but also to the extent of requiring that children should not be left unvaccinated. It has interfered between employer and employed, to the extent of insisting, in the interests of the latter, that certain sanitary claims shall be fulfilled in all places of industrial occupation. It has interfered between vendor and purchaser; has put restrictions on the sale and purchase of poisons, has prohibited in certain cases certain commercial supplies of water, and has made it a public offence to sell adulterated food or drink or medicine, or to offer for sale any meat unfit for human food. Its care for the treatment of disease has not been unconditionally limited to treating at the public expense such sickness as may accompany destitution: it has provided that in any sort of epidemic emergency organized medical assistance, not peculiarly for paupers, may be required of local authorities; and in the same spirit it

requires that vaccination at the public cost shall be given gratuitously to every claimant. [47]

From these public health developments it might seem that medicine was coming into its own, a knight in shining armour rescuing Britannia from the dragons of filth, cholera, environmental pollution, food adulteration and all the other health hazards produced by rampant population growth and unregulated *laissez faire*. At last, the nation (it seemed) had recognised the true worth of the medical profession. Yet – and this is a second paradox – that is not what happened.

For the organised medical profession played a surprisingly secondary and desultory role in the vast expansion of Victorian state health provision. Of course the work of hundreds of enlightened, humane practitioners throughout the nation in spotlighting the relations between squalor and disease cannot be gainsaid. In Manchester, for example, James Kay-Shuttleworth proved an indefatigable activist, publishing in 1832 his classic *The Moral and Physical Condition of the Working Classes* [26; 70]. Nevertheless, the Medical Colleges never gave an impetus to the public health movement; similarly the pages of the *Lancet* echoed with the internal political squabbles of the profession more than with campaigns to improve the people's health. Above all, neither of the two most vociferous public champions of health, Edwin Chadwick and Florence Nightingale – both determined and immensely long-lived – was a doctor. That was of course true of Miss Nightingale by definition, because the medical profession's restrictive practices debarred women from medicine until the 1870s. For his part, Chadwick was trained in the law, was a bureaucrat by temperament, and – perhaps most importantly – had done a stint as Jeremy Bentham's secretary [27; 49].

Moreover these great champions of public health were not only *not* doctors; they were in important ways positively anti-doctor. Chadwick in particular characterised the profession as supine and venal – a body with such a vested interest in disease as to lack motivation for its eradication. For him the profession's primary involvement with clinical medicine, with pathology, with treatment, put the cart before the horse. Prevention was better than cure (not, thought Chadwick, that doctors were very good at curing, in any case!). And prevention could not be achieved simply by individuals taking good care of themselves through diet, regimen and so on when they were, perforce, living in a lethal environment [62; 63].

Chadwick, Nightingale and their supporters offered alternative packages of theories of health and disease. Chadwick liked to represent the medical profession as committed to the 'contagionist' theory, i.e. the view that disease is spread through the transfer of disease 'seeds' by personal contact (a kind of precursor of Pasteur's germ theory). For Chadwick and like-minded sanitarians this was nonsense, for how was it that in epidemics, all people did not thereby 'catch' the disease? Instead Chadwick championed 'anti-contagionism' (as did a fair portion of doctors too), the view that sickness sprang from pestiferous 'miasmas', or contaminated atmospheres. Miasmas were bred and emitted by polluted water, sewage, animal ordure, industrial waste and the like: in his pithy dictum, 'all smell is disease' [17; 68].

From this it followed that securing the public health hardly needed the mysterious art of the clinician. Rather, towns had to be cleaned up. For Chadwick and his supporters this meant providing two things: a plentiful pure-water supply, both for drinking and for flushing away waste, and a system of underground mains-drainage, to ensure that waste really was flushed out of towns (down to the sea or to sewage farms) before it bred pestilence. So, public health was a matter of engineering not medicine. In the mid-Victorian era, miracles of civil engineering set up the water and drainage system for London which basically still works. Other towns followed suit. The death rate dropped: the doctors remained bystanders. The relative indifference of the medical establishment to preventive (as distinct from curative) medicine and to environmental and occupational medicine is one legacy we still have with us today [80].

6 The Role of Medicine: What Did it Achieve?

IN the last two chapters the rise of the medical profession has been traced from its comparatively restricted status in Tudor and Stuart times. From the eighteenth century, it shared in the general expansion of a market economy. In the nineteenth century it achieved public blessing as a liberal profession, and benefited from the state's growing involvement in public health.

But if medicine grew healthy, did it actually promote health in others? After all, George Bernard Shaw in his play, *The Doctor's Dilemma* (1906), could still present a bevy of top doctors shamelessly admitting to themselves that their medicine was essentially bogus. If Muggleton could opine in the seventeenth century, 'if there were never a doctor of physick in the world, people would live longer and live better in health', was such a view still tenable during the reign of Victoria? [93] And, if so, how then do we explain its persistence?

The grandest context in which to evaluate these questions is to ask whether medicine (from self-help to pukka physic, with public health thrown in as well) kept people alive: did it have any significant effect upon the aggregate population? The death rate was strikingly high through most of the seventeenth century, peaking again in the 1720s and 30s, declining somewhat from the 1740s, rising again during the early nineteenth-century decades of rapid industrialisation, and beginning a slow but sustained decline from around 1830, plummeting only in this century. Life expectancy, perhaps around 35 for males in the mid seventeenth century, was around 40 by 1850 and had risen to 44 by 1890 [28; 106].

The peaks and plateaux in the death rate were essentially due to 'mortality crises' caused by waves of epidemic disease, local or national, sporadic or sustained. Other major causes of death, such as famine, important elsewhere in Europe, disappeared in England [2].

So the question is: when the death rate dipped, did medicine play a key role? Or, more positively: did it have a part in the vast rise in population gathering momentum from the 1740s and lasting throughout the period covered in this survey and beyond?

Today's leading historical demographers have argued convincingly that this sustained population growth stemmed primarily from a rising birth rate, not from a falling death rate. In its turn, the rising birth rate is to be explained less by factors biological or medical than by social changes, above all, a trend towards earlier marriage amongst labouring people in an expansive economy full of opportunity and – as, say, in modern India – insecurity [106].

Yet still that leaves the question of the possible role of medicine in bringing down mortality. There is scant evidence that medicine could do much throughout this entire period to counter the great lethal diseases. The plague was not conquered; it disappeared from Britain after 1666, but this had nothing to do with medicine, something to do with quarantine as imposed on a European scale [87], but probably more to do with the mysteries of the epidemiology of rats and fleas. The same applies to cholera in the nineteenth century. It came, it conquered, it receded (possibly cleaner towns and water supplies had some impact) [25; 68]. Epidemics of typhus and dysentery caused mortality crises in the 1720s and 30s: fevers seem to have proved less lethal in subsequent decades, possibly because immunity had been acquired, but not because of any medical break-throughs. Not until the coming of antibiotics in the 1940s did medicine possess the power reliably to save victims of infectious diseases from death [21]. In 1694 Queen Mary died of smallpox. As late as 1861, no less a personage than Prince Albert succumbed to typhoid.

Indeed, a distinguished medical professor, Thomas McKeown, has gone so far as to question 'the role of medicine' even in the very real and continued fall in the death rate, a fall that accelerated during Victoria's reign. Death claimed fewer victims, McKeown argues, not because medicine improved (hospitals, he thinks, 'positively did harm'), but mainly because of improved nutrition, made possible by a rising standard of living, which increased the nation's resistance. The environmental clean-up also played its part, McKeown believes [55].

The contrast McKeown draws between the roles of medicine and of engineering and nutrition is too extreme and artificial; and the current verdict upon hospitals is now more favourable (if they had really been 'gateways to death', it is hard to see why community and doctors alike continued to patronise them) [105]. But, applied to the period from c. 1650 to c. 1850, his basic scepticism about medicine holds good. Medicine succeeded in making only marginal inroads into fatal diseases. It scored one notable triumph. Between them, smallpox inoculation (introduced, be it remembered, by a lay woman) and vaccination (the work of Edward Jenner, a country doctor) diminished the terrors of a once-prevalent and commonly fatal disease, and so made some demographic contribution, not least because smallpox commonly left its survivors sterile. But what Razzell has called 'the conquest of smallpox' was matched by no equivalent conquest [76]. Medical science made its advances, Harvey discovered the circulation of the blood, William Hunter explained the lymphatic system, the workings of the nervous system were revealed, the physiology of respiration and digestion understood; but these advances in basic medical science could not be translated into therapeutic weapons, not least because the causes of disease and the nature of the body's morbid responses remained deeply obscure and much contested. Advances in pathological anatomy, in cell science, basic physiology and organic chemistry, and the systematic observation of the sick *en masse* in hospitals did not bear significant fruit for saving lives till beyond the period covered by this survey. Modern surgery could not develop before the combination of anaesthetics and antiseptic (and later aseptic) conditions pioneered by Lister and others in the 1860s. The fall in the death rate from the 1820s is hard to explain with confidence. It may have something to do with the life-cycle of infectious diseases. From about mid century, however, better living standards and nutrition and improved sanitary conditions must take much credit [4; 6].

Does this mean that medicine was and remained Shaw's 'conspiracy', or at best a placebo offering psychological solace and hope (even if false hope) to those it could not offer cures? Of course one should not despise the role of the doctor as drug, if that role was well played. In a society in which for complex reasons the Christian clergy were ceasing to meet the personal needs of many – a society in which other comfort-giving professionals, such as social workers and psychiatric personnel, had not yet emerged – the trusted family doctor had much to contribute, through the confidences of the sick-bed, as friend, advisor and guide. Eighteenth- and nineteenth-century letters, diaries and fiction show that many practitioners were indeed admired and respected in such roles. The family doctor frequently became a valued arbitrator and authority in domestic discord. Such authority might of course be double-edged. The doctor's say might convince a husband that it would be medically unwise for his wife to get pregnant again. On the other hand, as feminist scholars have rightly insisted, male-dominated medicine itself helped reinforce a vision of women as the weaker sex, incapable of responsibilities, exertion or even serious education, fit only for motherhood and domesticity. This vision blighted the lives of so many Victorian women [78].

But medicine was in fact far more than a placebo, or just a bedside manner. It could not vanquish the fatal diseases, but it could reduce pain, palliate discomfort, patch people up, and help them to cope with chronic disorders and disabilities – leg ulcers, abscesses, rheumatism, gout, dyspepsia and so forth. True, what the doctor ordered was often little different from what common sense dictated. Gout sufferers discovered for themselves that they hit the bottle at their peril. But the good clinician knew by training and experience how to manage conditions such as dropsy – severe and painful, though rarely immediately fatal – which might be beyond the know-how of the layman. Similarly, he was a valuable surgeon who could set a fracture cleanly, or deliver a malpresented baby which had thwarted nature and baffled the midwife's art.

This was the human face of medicine. But was it, as an organised profession, more sinister? Radicals such as Ivan Illich have argued that medicine today is indeed a conspiracy, in that it 'expropriates' health management from the people to the doctors, and 'medicalizes' life, in the sense of claiming that many of the decisions about how we should run our affairs should be resolved only by medical experts [41]. Moreover, it is a 'con', argues Illich, because it allegedly creates more sickness than it cures.

Whatever the situation today, such an analysis hardly applies to early modern, or even early industrial times. The medical profession had not enveigled itself far into public life. It did not command a monopoly: it held few legal privileges: it was divided against itself. Unlike the other traditional professions – the law, the church, the army – it was hardly an arm of state. And not least, lay medicine and client control of doctors remained widespread. Without the confident power of being able to conquer disease and tame death – a power that did not emerge till the present century – the doctor's place in society necessarily remained ambiguous.

Select Bibliography

[1] Abel-Smith, Brian, *The Hospitals, 1800–1914* (London: Heinemann, 1964). A valuable survey, though concentrating mainly on administration and organisation.

[2] Appleby, A.B., *Famine in Tudor and Stuart England* (Liverpool: Liverpool University Press, 1978). Convincingly shows that mortality crises in seventeenth-century England were not a function of mass starvation, unlike through much of the Continent.

[3] Black, W.G., *Folk Medicine: a chapter in the history of culture* (London: Publications of the Folk-Lore Society, 1883). Though outmoded in its assumptions, this remains a major sourcebook for the dimensions of popular medicine.

[4] Buer, M.C., *Health, Wealth, and Population in the Early Days of the Industrial Revolution* (London: G. Routledge & Sons, 1926). Despite its superseded demographic data, contains valuable discussion of eighteenth-century steps in the directions of public health and hygiene.

[5] Burnby, J.G.L., 'A Study of the English Apothecary from 1660 to 1760', *Medical History*, Supplement 3 (1983). Presents abundant data to demonstrate that apothecaries existed in substantial numbers and shared advances in prosperity.

[6] Burnett, J., *Plenty and Want: A Social History of Diet in England from 1815 to the Present Day* (London: Nelson, 1966). Highly readable survey of diet, in the context of changing standards of living, and its implications for health.

[7] Bynum, W.F. and Porter, Roy (eds), *Williams Hunter and the Eighteenth Century Medical World* (Cambridge: Cambridge University Press, 1985). Explorations of the world of London medicine in the eighteenth century, including discussions of career structures, man-midwifery and medical education.

[8] Bynum, W.F. and Porter, Roy (eds), *Medical Fringe and Medical Orthodoxy 1750–1850* (London: Croom Helm, 1986). Analyses the changing relations between regular and irregular medicine in context of medical professionalisation and the state.

[9] Cameron, H.C., *Mr Guy's Hospital, 1726–1948* (London, New York and Toronto: Longmans Green, 1954). Brings out the importance of individual philanthropy in the development of the English hospital system.

[10] Cartwright, F.F., *A Social History of Medicine* (London: Longman, 1977). Though highly compressed and selective, this represents the best attempt yet to place medical transformations in their social context.

[11] [Chadwick, Edwin], *The Poor Law Report of 1834*, S.G. and O.A. Checkland (eds) (Harmondsworth: Penguin, 1974). The most influential official publication for changing attitudes on public health published in the nineteenth century, reprinted with a useful introduction.

[12] Chapman, Stanley, *Jesse Boot of Boots the Chemists* (London: Hodder & Stoughton, 1973). Demonstrates how Boots the Chemists had its origins in the Victorian medical fringe.

[13] Clark, Sir George, *A History of the Royal College of Physicians of London*, 3 vols (Oxford: Clarendon Press, 1964, 1966, 1972). The standard official history of the College, packed with facts, rather bland in tone.

[14] Clark-Kennedy, Archibald E., *London Pride: The story of a voluntary hospital* (London: Hutchinson Benham, 1979). A well-researched account of the London, one of the new voluntary hospitals of the Georgian age.

[15] Clarkson, Leslie, *Death, Disease and Famine in Pre-Industrial England* (Dublin: Gill and Macmillan, 1975). Illuminating analysis of the interplay between social and biological forces in the patterns of morbidity and mortality, valuable for making sense of more strictly demographic sources, such as [106].

[16] Cook, Harold J., *The Decline of the Old Medical Regime in Stuart London* (Ithaca: Cornell University Press, 1986). Examines the politics of London medicine in the seventeenth century, especially the declining fortunes of the College of Physicians. Good counterbalance to Webster [99].

[17] Cooter, R., 'Anticontagionism and History's Medical

Record', in P. Wright and A. Treacher (eds), *The Problem of Medical Knowledge* (Edinburgh: Edinburgh University Press, 1982), pp. 87–108. Illuminating exploration of how theories of disease were deeply involved with social, moral and political attitudes.

[18] Cope, Sir Zachary, 'The Private Medical Schools of London 1746–1914', in Poynter, F.N.L. (ed.), *The Evolution of Medical Education in Britain* (London: Pitman, 1966), pp. 89–109. Shows the important role which private institutions played in the rise of English medical education.

[19] Cope, Sir Vincent Zachary, *The History of the Royal College of Surgeons of England* (London: Anthony Blond, 1959). Useful, but 'official' in its outlooks. The College requires fresh historical interpretation.

[20] Copeman, W.S.C., *The Worshipful Society of Apothecaries of London. A History 1617–1967* (Oxford: Pergamon Press, 1967). Correctly emphasises the role of the Society as a trade guild.

[21] Creighton, Charles, *A History of Epidemics in Britain* (Cambridge, Cambridge University Press), 2 vols [1891–4]. New Edition 1965. A massive compilation, unreliable in its details, but still of great value for its quantity of evidence.

[22] Dainton, Courtney, *The Story of England's Hospitals* (London: Museum Press, 1961). In the absence of any full scholarly survey of the rise of hospitals, this rather slight work still has some value.

[23] Digby, Anne, *Madness, Morality and Medicine. A Study of the York Retreat, 1796–1914* (Cambridge: Cambridge University Press, 1985). Fully-researched and penetrating analysis of the workings of England's leading private lunatic asylum, especially welcome for its emphasis upon the patients.

[24] Donnison, Jean, *Midwives and Medical Men: A history of interprofessional rivalries and women's rights* (London: Heinemann Educational, 1977). A powerfully written account of how men came to replace women from the late seventeenth century onwards as the providers of obstetrical services.

[25] Durey, M., *The Return of the Plague: British Society and the Cholera 1831–2* (Dublin: Gill and Macmillan, 1979). Excellent for the social, moral and political responses to cholera.

[26] Eyler, J.M., *Victorian Social Medicine. The Ideas and Methods*

of William Farr (Baltimore: Johns Hopkins University Press, 1979). An intelligent and sympathetic intellectual biography of the leading medical statistician of Victorian England, showing how data helped waken the public conscience.

[27] Finer, S.E., *Life and Times of Edwin Chadwick* (London: Methuen, 1952). Superb biography of the leading public health campaigner, with an intelligent assessment of the importance of Chadwick's utilitarian background.

[28] Flinn, Michael W., *The European Demographic System 1500–1820* (Brighton, Sussex, Harvester Press, 1981). Powerful overview of how Europe as a whole broke out of the biological 'ancien regime'. Good on comparative themes.

[29] Fraser, D., *The Evolution of the British Welfare State. A History of Social Policy since the Industrial Revolution* (London: Macmillan, 1973). A well-digested and balanced survey of the growing role of the state in providing public health and welfare. Sensitive to alternative interpretations.

[30] Frazer, W.M., *A History of English Public Health, 1834–1939* (London; Baillière, 1950). A solid, factual account.

[31] Gitting, Clare, *Death, Burial and the Individual in Early Modern England* (London: Croom Helm, 1984). Provides lots of insights into attitudes towards death, which the author sees as an increasingly 'individual' experience.

[32] Green, David G., *Working Class Patients and the Medical Establishment. Self Help in Britain from the mid nineteenth century to 1948* (London: Gower/Maurice Temple Smith, 1985). An admiring exploration of the health provisions of friendly societies.

[33] Hamilton, B., 'The Medical Professions in the Eighteenth Century', *Economic History Review*, 2nd series, IV (1951), 141–69. Though dated, still a valuable account of the structuring of the medical professions. Use together with the work of Lane, Loudon and Waddington.

[34] Hamilton, D., *The Healers: A history of medicine in Scotland* (Edinburgh: Canongate, 1981). Brings out the special contribution of the Scots to British medicine, in particular the scientific education provided from early times by Edinburgh and then Glasgow universities.

[35] Helman, Cecil, *Culture, Health and Illness* (Bristol: John Wright, 1984). Stimulating and imaginative exploration of the

meanings of health and disease, and the symbolic significance of therapies, from the viewpoint of the sick person and the community.

[36] Hobhouse, Edmund, *The Dairy of a West Country Physician, AD 1684-1726* (London: Simpkin Marshall, 1934). Reveals the medical practice of Claver Morris, a practitioner from Wells.

[37] Hodgkinson, Ruth G., *The Origins of the National Health Service: The medical services of the new Poor Law, 1834–1871* (Wellcome Historical Medical Library, London, 1967). Very fully documented account of the rise of the Poor Law medical service, following the New Poor Law of 1834.

[38] Holloway, S.W.F., 'Medical Education in England, 1830–1858: A Sociological Analysis', *History*, XLIX (1964), 299–324. Demonstrates that debates over the quality of medical education reflected deep divisions within the medical profession about its own structure.

[39] Holloway, S.W.F., 'The Apothecaries' Act of 1815: A Reinterpretation', 2 parts, *Medical History*, 10:2 (1966), 107–29; and 10:3 (1966), 221–36. A major revisionist piece, arguing that the apothecaries probably lost more than they gained by the Act of 1815, and thus showing the strength of the old hierarchy.

[40] Hultin, N.C., 'Medicine and Magic in the Eighteenth Century: the Diaries of James Woodforde', *Journal of the History of Medicine and Allied Sciences*, 30 (1975), 349–66. Fascinating account of the 'magical' remedies used by the mid-eighteenth-century parson.

[41] Illich, I., *The Limits of Medicine* (Harmondsworth: Penguin Books, 1978). Primarily a polemic, though with a historical dimension, denouncing the alleged rise of modern dependency upon medicine, and the medical profession's part in fostering that dependence.

[42] Inglis, Brian, *Fringe Medicine* (London: Faber & Faber, 1964). An enterprising attempt to trace the roots of the modern medical fringe. Use in connection with [8].

[43] Jewson, N., 'Medical Knowledge and the Patronage System in Eighteenth Century England', *Sociology*, XII (1974), 369–85. Argues rather schematically that traditional medicine, both as social practice and as scientific theory, depended heavily upon the influence wielded by aristocratic patients.

[44] Johnson, T.J., *Professions and Power* (London and Basingstoke: Macmillan, 1972). Argues against the 'altruistic' view of professions, seeing them as concerned to gain quasi-monopolistic powers for their members.

[45] Jones, Kathleen, *A History of the Mental Health Services* (London and Boston: Routledge & Kegan Paul, 1972). Important if rather idealistic account of the state's growing involvement with mental health.

[46] Keevil, J.J., *Medicine and the Navy 1200–1900*, 2 vols (vol. 1, 1200–1649, vol. 2, 1649–1714) (Edinburgh and London: Livingstone, 1957–63). A massive and well-documented history. See also [50].

[47] Lambert, R., *Sir John Simon 1816–1904 and English Social Administration* (London: MacGibbon and Kee, 1963). The authoritative biography of the most important medical officer of the state in the nineteenth century.

[48] Lane, Joan, 'The Medical Practitioners of Provincial England in 1783', *Medical History*, xxviii (1984), 353–71. Important analysis of the structure of provincial practice in the late eighteenth century.

[49] Lewis, R.A., *Edwin Chadwick and the Public Health Movement 1832–1854* (London: Longmans Green, 1952). Relates Chadwick's life to the growing public concern about health matters.

[50] Lloyd, C. and Coulter, J.S.L., *Medicine and the Navy 1200–1900* (vol. 3, 1714–1815, vol. 4, 1815–1900) (Edinburgh and London: Livingstone, 1961–3). A massive and standard history. See also [46].

[51] Loudon, Irvine S., 'The Origins and Growth of the Dispensary Movement in England', *Bulletin of the History of Medicine*, iv (1981), 322–42. Examines the dispensary movement as one of the roots of public health concern.

[52] Loudon, Irvine S., *Medical Care and the General Practitioner, 1750–1850* (Oxford: Oxford University Press, 1987). A fundamentally important account of the emergence of the family doctor.

[53] McClure, Ruth, *Coram's Children* (New Haven, Connecticut, and London: Yale University Press, 1981). A well-researched account of London's main orphanage, arguing that it was efficiently and humanely managed.

[54] McGrew, Roderick E., *Encyclopedia of Medical History* (London: Macmillan, 1985). A reliable reference work on the history of medical theory and practice.

[55] McKeown, Thomas, *The Modern Rise of Population* (London: Edward Arnold, 1976). McKeown casts doubt on the idea that medical progress produced diminished mortality. Nutrition and environmental factors instead are stressed.

[56] McLaren, A., *Reproductive Rituals* (New York: Methuen, 1984). A pioneering survey of popular attitudes and practices with regard to pregnancy, reproduction and infanticide.

[57] Matthews, Leslie G., *History of Pharmacy in Britain* (Edinburgh and London: Livingstone, 1962). Useful narrative account.

[58] Miller, G., *The Adoption of Inoculation for Smallpox in England and France* (London: Oxford University Press, 1957). Shows the importance of social and political factors in the faster adoption of inoculation in Britain.

[59] Morris, R.J., *Cholera, 1832* (London: Croom Helm, 1976). Is particularly interesting on the relative impact – physically and mentally – of cholera on different classes of society.

[60] Mullett, Charles, 'Public baths and health in England, 16th–18th century', *Bulletin of the History of Medicine*, Supplement No. 5 (Baltimore, 1946). By showing the relative importance of public baths, Mullett undermines the popular notion that cleanliness was a nineteenth-century invention.

[61] Newman, Charles, *The Evolution of Medical Education in the 19th century* (London: Oxford University Press, 1957). The standard history of the emergence of the modern teaching hospital.

[62] Newman, George, *The Rise of Preventive Medicine* (Oxford/London: Oxford University Press, 1932). Surveys the concept of prevention from Antiquity onwards.

[63] Newsholme, Sir Arthur, *Evolution of Preventive Medicine* (Baltimore: Williams & Wilkins, 1927). Though dated, contains an important insider's account of the role increasingly played by the state in public health.

[64] Owen, David, *English Philanthropy 1660–1940* (Cambridge, Massachusetts: Belknap Press, 1965). Demonstrates the importance of charity and humanitarianism in the growth of medical facilities in England.

[65] Oxley, G.W., *Poor Relief in England and Wales 1601–1834* (Newton Abbot: David and Charles, 1974). A clear, brief guide to the workings of the Old Poor Law.

[66] Parry, Noel and Parry, Jose, *The Rise of the Medical Profession. A Study of Collective Social Mobility* (London: Croom Helm, 1976). A sociological perspective on the rise of the modern medical profession.

[67] Parry-Jones, William, *The Trade in Lunacy. A Study of Private Madhouses in England in the Eighteenth and Nineteenth Centuries* (London: Routledge & Kegan Paul, 1972). Shows, through a wealth of detail, the importance of private provision in the emergence of care for the mad.

[68] Pelling, M., *Cholera, Fever and English Medicine 1825–1865* (Oxford: Oxford University Press, 1978). Particularly strong on the alternative medical theories for understanding and combating cholera.

[69] Peterson, M.J., *The Medical Profession in Mid-Victorian London* (Berkeley: University of California Press, 1978). The best account of the emergence of the modern British medical profession, stressing the importance of specialisation, the teaching hospitals and the rise of Harley Street.

[70] Pickstone, John V., *Medicine and Industrial Society. A History of Hospital Development in Manchester and its Region 1752–1946* (Manchester: Manchester University Press, 1985). A major account of the place played by voluntary and municipal hospitals in the life of new industrial communities.

[71] Porter, Roy (ed.), *Patients and Practitioners. Lay Perceptions of Medicine in Pre-Industrial Society* (Cambridge: Cambridge University Press, 1985). Essays examining how sick people coped with disease and with their doctors.

[72] Porter, Roy, 'The Patient's View: Doing Medical History from Below', *Theory and Society*, XIV (1985), 175–98. States the priorities of a patient-centred social history of medicine.

[73] Pound, Reginald, *Harley Street* (London: Michael Joseph, 1967). Anecdotal but informative.

[74] Poynter, F.N.L. (ed.), *The Evolution of Medical Education in Britain* (London: Pitman, 1966). Essays looking at the variety of forms of medical education, including apprenticeship.

[75] Poynter, F.N.L. (ed.), *The Evolution of Hospitals in Britain*

(London, Pitman, 1964). Essays examining the diverse forms of hospital provision in England, both public and private, general and specialised.

[76] Razzell, Peter, *The Conquest of Smallpox* (Firle, Sussex: Caliban Press, 1975). Argues that the work of Jenner has been misinterpreted and overrated, and shows that inoculation was relatively safe and an important life-saver.

[77] Roberts, David, *Victorian Origins of the British Welfare State* (New Haven: Yale University Press, 1960). Broad and sympathetic account of state intervention in the Victorian age.

[78] Roberts, R. (ed.), *Women, Health and Reproduction* (London: Routledge & Kegan Paul, 1981). Essays mainly from a feminist point of view, showing that the rise of modern, male-dominated medicine is a mixed blessing for women.

[79] Roberts, R.S., 'The Personnel and Practice of Medicine in Tudor and Stuart England', *Medical History*, vi (1962), 363–82; vii (1964), 217–34. A pioneer survey. Use with [98].

[80] Rosen, George, *A History of Public Health* (New York: MD Publications, 1958). The major broad survey of the history of public health on an international plane.

[81] Russell, Andrew W. (ed.), *The Town and State Physician in Europe from the Middle Ages to the Enlightenment* (Wolfenbüttel: Herzog August Bibliothek, 1981). Essays examining the civic roots of the public health movement in many European countries.

[82] Schupbach, William, 'Sequah: An English "American Medicine-Man" in 1890', *Medical History*, xxix (1985), 272–317. Vivid account of a late nineteenth-century quack.

[83] Sheppard, F., *London, 1808–1870: the Infernal Wen* (London: Secker & Warburg, 1971). Detailed account of the health problems of a rapidly expanding metropolis.

[84] Shorter, Edward, *A History of Women's Bodies* (London: Allen Lane, 1982). A controversial history which seeks to establish the benefits which modern medicine has brought to women, in particular through reducing childbirth mortality.

[85] Shorter, Edward, *Bedside Manners* (Harmondsworth: Allen Lane, 1986). A brisk history, covering America, Britain and Europe, of the changing status of the general practitioner.

[86] Slack, Paul, 'Books of Orders: The making of English social policy, 1577–1631', *Transactions of the Royal Historical*

Society, 5th Series, 30 (1980) 1–22. Examines provision for health as part of a broader emergence of social policy.

[87] Slack, Paul, *The Impact of Plague in Tudor and Stuart England* (London: Routledge & Kegan Paul, 1985). A major account of responses, political, social, medical and religious, to the great scourge of the sixteenth and seventeenth centuries. Argues that more effective measures slowly emerged.

[88] Smith, F.B., *The People's Health 1830–1910* (London: Croom Helm, 1979). Statistically-rich investigation of the state of the nation's health in the nineteenth century; short on interpretation.

[89] Sprigge, S. Squire, *The Life and Times of Thomas Wakley, Founder and First Editor of the 'Lancet', Member of Parliament for Finsbury and Coroner for West Middlesex* (London: Longmans, Green and Co., 1899). The best biography of one of the key medical campaigners and reformers of the nineteenth century.

[90] Starr, P., *The Social Transformation of American Medicine* (New York: Basic Books, 1982). A sociologically-oriented interpretation of the changing place of doctors in American society.

[91] Thane, P., *The Foundations of the Welfare State* (London: Longman, 1982). Clear and balanced account.

[92] Thomas, E.G., 'The Old Poor Law and Medicine', *Medical History*, xxiv (1980), 1–19. Shows that the Old Poor Law was quite generous in its medical provisions.

[93] Thomas, Keith, *Religion and the Decline of Magic. Studies in Popular Beliefs in Sixteenth- and Seventeenth-Century England* (London: Weidenfeld and Nicolson, 1971). Contains a wealth of material on popular medicine and its connections to magic and witchcraft.

[94] Turner, E.S., *Call the Doctor: A Social History of Medical Men* (London: Michael Joseph, 1958). A lively, popular narrative.

[95] Versluysen, Margaret Connor, 'Midwives, Medical men and "Poor Women Labouring of Child"; Lying-in Hospitals in Eighteenth Century London', in H. Roberts (ed.), *Women, Health and Reproduction* (London: Routledge & Kegan Paul, 1981), pp. 18–49. Important interpretation of the effects for

women of the emergence of maternity hospitals in the eighteenth century.

[96] Waddington, Ivan, 'The Struggle to Reform the Royal College of Physicians, 1767–1771: A Sociological Analysis', *Medical History*, xvii (1973), 107–26. Demonstrates how successfully entrenched the existing medical hierarchy was.

[97] Waddington, Ivan, *The Medical Profession in the Industrial Revolution* (Dublin: Gill and Macmillan, 1984). A mature and well-organised account of the 'modernization' of the medical profession, discounting any simple theory of 'progress'.

[98] Webster, Charles (ed.), *Health, Medicine and Mortality in the Sixteenth Century* (Cambridge: Cambridge University Press, 1979). Essays full of informative research relating to the early modern medical profession.

[99] Webster, Charles, *The Great Instauration. Science, Medicine and Reform, 1626–1660* (London: Duckworth, 1975). The best account of attempts (mainly 'Puritan') to reform medicine in the seventeenth century, showing how the Restoration of 1660 spelt their failure.

[100] Weindling, Paul (ed.), *The Social History of Occupational Health* (London: Croom Helm, 1985). A major account of job-related disease and the rise of occupational medicine.

[101] Williams, G., *The Age of Miracles. Medicine and Surgery in the Nineteenth Century* (London: Constable, 1981). A popular history of nineteenth-century medicine.

[102] Williams, G., *The Age of Agony: The Art of Healing c. 1700–1800* (London: Constable, 1975). A popular account of eighteenth-century medicine.

[103] Wohl, A.S., *The Eternal Slum. Housing and Social Policy in Victorian London* (London: Edward Arnold, 1977). Shows how revelations of unhealthy living conditions led to urban reform.

[104] Wohl, Anthony S., *Endangered Lives. Public Health in Victorian Britain* (London: Dent, 1983). A fine analysis of the part played by medical men in the generation of public health agitation.

[105] Woodward, John, *To Do the Sick No Harm. A Study of the British Voluntary Hospital System to 1875* (London and Boston: Routledge & Kegan Paul, 1974) (International

Library of Social Policy, ed. Kathleen Jones). A valuable history of the voluntary hospital movement.

[106] Wrigley, E.A. and Schofield, R.S., *The Population History of England, 1541–1871. A Reconstruction* (London: Edward Arnold, 1981). The standard source for English demographic history, though it has relatively little to say on the medical dimensions of morbidity and mortality.

Additional Bibliography

[107] Woods, Robert and Woodward, John, *Urban Disease and Mortality in Nineteenth Century England* (London: Batsford, 1984). Valuable essays integrating urban history, historical demography and medical history.

[108] Riley, James C., *The Eighteenth-Century Campaign to Avoid Disease* (London: Macmillan, 1986). Important new study of early preventive medicine.

Index

anaesthetics, 63
antiseptics, 63
apothecaries, 19, 34
Apothecaries, Society of, 19, 51;
    Apothecaries Act (1815), 49
Arnold, Thomas, 43
asylums, 42

Bacon, Francis, 13
Baillie, Matthew, 39, 40
Barber Surgeons Company, 18
Baxter, Richard, 24, 28
Bentham, Jeremy and
    Benthamites, 56
Board of Health, 58
Boot, Jesse, 47
British Medical Association, 52,
    55

Chadwick, Edwin, 56, 59, 60
cholera, 57, 62
Contagious Diseases Act (1867),
    58

Darwin, Erasmus, 40
death, 27; death rate, 63–4
Dell, William, 13
Dimsdale, Thomas, 41
dispensaries, 37
drugs, 15

empirics, 20
epidemics, 26, 61, 62

Fothergill, John, 33

Galen, 13, 15
Garth, Samuel, 40
General Medical Council, 51
general practitioners, 34, 52–4,
    64
Greatrakes, Valentine, 21

Harvey, William, 32
Heberden, William, 39
herbalism, 46
hospitals, 22, 35–7, 62;
    maternity, 36
Howard, John, 55
humours, 25
Hunter, William, 33, 39, 40, 63

incomes, 40
inoculation, 41
insanity, 22

James, Robert, and his Fever
    Powders, 46
Jenner, Edward, 63
Johnson, Samuel, 30, 46
Josselin, Ralph, 20, 28

Kay-Shuttleworth, Sir James, 59

Lancet, The, 48
Lettsom, J. C., 33, 39
lunatic asylums, 36, 43